Evidence-Based Diagnosis and Management of Facial Nerve Disorders

Evidence-Based Diagnosis and Management of Facial Nerve Disorders

Editors

Gerd Fabian Volk
Steffen U. Eisenhardt
Shai M. Rozen

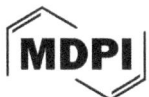

Basel • Beijing • Wuhan • Barcelona • Belgrade • Novi Sad • Cluj • Manchester

Editors
Gerd Fabian Volk
Jena University Hospital
Jena, Germany

Steffen U. Eisenhardt
Medical Center-University of Freiburg
Freiburg, Germany

Shai M. Rozen
University of Texas
Southwestern Medical Center
Dallas, TX, USA

Editorial Office
MDPI
St. Alban-Anlage 66
4052 Basel, Switzerland

This is a reprint of articles from the Special Issue published online in the open access journal *Diagnostics* (ISSN 2075-4418) (available at: https://www.mdpi.com/journal/diagnostics/special_issues/Facial_Nerve_Disord).

For citation purposes, cite each article independently as indicated on the article page online and as indicated below:

Lastname, A.A.; Lastname, B.B. Article Title. *Journal Name* **Year**, *Volume Number*, Page Range.

ISBN 978-3-0365-9390-6 (Hbk)
ISBN 978-3-0365-9391-3 (PDF)
doi.org/10.3390/books978-3-0365-9391-3

Cover image courtesy of Gerd Fabian Volk, painted by Christian Eisenberger 2019 (EIS/M 307): "The head is a general topic of mine. I make heads in series because a lot of things fail. This can lead to multiple failures."

© 2023 by the authors. Articles in this book are Open Access and distributed under the Creative Commons Attribution (CC BY) license. The book as a whole is distributed by MDPI under the terms and conditions of the Creative Commons Attribution-NonCommercial-NoDerivs (CC BY-NC-ND) license.

Contents

About the Editors vii

Gerd Fabian Volk, Caroline Cora Kraus, Steffen U. Eisenhardt and Shai Rozen
Special Issue: Evidence-Based Diagnosis and Management of Facial Nerve Disorders
Reprinted from: *Diagnostics* **2022**, *12*, 3056, doi:10.3390/diagnostics13193056 1

Hanna Rüschenschmidt, Gerd Fabian Volk, Christoph Anders and Orlando Guntinas-Lichius
Electromyography of Extrinsic and Intrinsic Ear Muscles in Healthy Probands and Patients with Unilateral Postparalytic Facial Synkinesis
Reprinted from: *Diagnostics* **2022**, *12*, 121, doi:10.3390/diagnostics12010121 3

Myung Chul Yoo
Diagnostic Value of Preoperative Electrodiagnostic Analysis in a Patient with Facial Palsy and a Large Vestibular Schwannoma: Case Report
Reprinted from: *Diagnostics* **2022**, *12*, 542, doi:10.3390/diagnostics12020542 13

Ciro Emiliano Boschetti, Giorgio Lo Giudice, Chiara Spuntarelli, Carmine Apice, Raffaele Rauso, Mario Santagata, et al.
Kabat Rehabilitation in Facial Nerve Palsy after Parotid Gland Tumor Surgery: A Case-Control Study
Reprinted from: *Diagnostics* **2022**, *12*, 565, doi:10.3390/diagnostics12030565 21

Florian Schmidt, Katy Bradley and Gerd Fabian Volk
Osteoradionecrosis of the Temporal Bone as a Rare Cause of Facial Nerve Palsy
Reprinted from: *Diagnostics* **2022**, *12*, 1021, doi:10.3390/diagnostics12051021 33

Anna-Maria Kuttenreich, Gerd Fabian Volk, Orlando Guntinas-Lichius, Harry von Piekartz and Stefan Heim
Facial Emotion Recognition in Patients with Post-Paralytic Facial Synkinesis—A Present Competence
Reprinted from: *Diagnostics* **2022**, *12*, 1138, doi:10.3390/diagnostics12051138 41

Helen Abing, Carina Pick, Tabea Steffens, Jenny Shachi Sharma, Jens Peter Klußmann and Maria Grosheva
Reanimation of the Smile with Neuro-Vascular Anastomosed Gracilis Muscle: A Case Series
Reprinted from: *Diagnostics* **2022**, *12*, 1282, doi:10.3390/diagnostics12051282 63

Gemma S. Parra-Dominguez, Carlos H. Garcia-Capulin and Raul E. Sanchez-Yanez
Automatic Facial Palsy Diagnosis as a Classification Problem Using Regional Information Extracted from a Photograph
Reprinted from: *Diagnostics* **2022**, *12*, 1528, doi:10.3390/diagnostics12071528 75

Andreas Kehrer, Marc Ruewe, Natascha Platz Batista da Silva, Daniel Lonic, Paul Immanuel Heidekrueger, Samuel Knoedler, et al.
Using High-Resolution Ultrasound to Assess Post-Facial Paralysis Synkinesis—Machine Settings and Technical Aspects for Facial Surgeons
Reprinted from: *Diagnostics* **2022**, *12*, 1650, doi:10.3390/diagnostics12071650 93

Anna-Maria Kuttenreich, Harry von Piekartz and Stefan Heim
Is There a Difference in Facial Emotion Recognition after Stroke with vs. without Central Facial Paresis?
Reprinted from: *Diagnostics* **2022**, *12*, 1721, doi:10.3390/diagnostics12071721 105

**Tsubasa Kitama, Makoto Hosoya, Masaru Noguchi, Takanori Nishiyama,
Takeshi Wakabayashi, Marie N. Shimanuki, et al.**
Intratemporal Facial Nerve Schwannomas: A Review of 45 Cases in A Single Center
Reprinted from: *Diagnostics* **2022**, *12*, 1789, doi:10.3390/diagnostics12081789 127

Charles Nduka, Ruben Yap Kannan, Gerd Fabian Volk and Orlando Guntinas-Lichius
Comment on Kehrer et al. Using High-Resolution Ultrasound to Assess Post-Facial Paralysis Synkinesis—Machine Settings and Technical Aspects for Facial Surgeons. *Diagnostics* 2022, *12*, 1650
Reprinted from: *Diagnostics* **2022**, *12*, 2431, doi:10.3390/diagnostics12102431 135

Andreas Kehrer, Lukas Prantl, Samuel Knoedler and Leonard Knoedler
Reply to Nduka et al. Comment on "Kehrer et al. Using High-Resolution Ultrasound to Assess Post-Facial Paralysis Synkinesis—Machine Settings and Technical Aspects for Facial Surgeons. *Diagnostics* 2022, *12*, 1650"
Reprinted from: *Diagnostics* **2022**, *12*, 2432, doi:10.3390/diagnostics12102432 137

About the Editors

Gerd Fabian Volk

Gerd Fabian Volk (PD Dr. med. Habil.): Gerd Fabian Volk has been active since 2006 as a physician at the Department of Otorhinolaryngology of Jena University Hospital. Since 2012, he has been the leader of the interdisciplinary Facial-Nerve-Center Jena. His clinical interests are as follows: the diagnosis and treatment of facial nerve palsy, telemedicine to improve the diagnosis and treatment of rare diseases, application of botulinum toxin and electrostimulation in the head and neck region, functional diagnostics and therapy of peripheral nerve lesions, and electrophysiological and imaging techniques for the evaluation and rehabilitation of the muscles and nerves. Experimental topics include the following: the development of new methods of reconstruction of the facial and laryngeal nerve; electrostimulation as a diagnostic and therapeutic tool; central changes after brain nerve failure, in particular of the facial and vestibular nerves; and telemedicine and health care networks to improve treatment quality.

Steffen U. Eisenhardt

Steffen U. Eisenhardt (Prof. Dr. med.), Steffen U. Eisenhardt is a plastic and reconstructive surgeon with over 15 years of experience. He is a member of the German Society for Plastic, Reconstructive and Aesthetic Surgeons (DGPRÄC), the German Society for Microcirculation and Vascular Biology (GfMVB) and the European Plastic Surgery Research Council. In 1998, he began his medical studies at University of Freiburg and is now full professor and head of Department of Plastic and Handsurgery at University of Freiburg Medical Center. His research focuses on innate immunity, innate memory, immunology of allotransplant rejection, "liquid biopsy" and tumor markers in soft tissue sarcomas.

Shai M. Rozen

Shai M. Rozen (M.D.), Shai M. Rozen is a Professor in the Department of Plastic Surgery at UT Southwestern Medical Center. He specializes in facial paralysis correction surgery and breast reconstruction.

Dr. Rozen earned his medical degree at the Tel Aviv University Sackler School of Medicine. He completed separate residencies first in general surgery and then in plastic surgery at Johns Hopkins Hospital in Baltimore. He then received advanced training in craniofacial surgery through a fellowship at the International Craniofacial Institute, followed by extensive training in peripheral nerve surgery through a fellowship at Johns Hopkins.

He joined the UT Southwestern faculty in 2007.

At UT Southwestern, he has co-created with colleagues from otolaryngology and neurosurgery a specialty group treating patients with facial paralysis. In addition, he treats patients with significant facial deformities and breast cancer patients in need of breast reconstruction using microsurgical techniques. He also treats a unique group of patients with pain situations stemming from nerve injuries. His cosmetic specialization is in the areas in which he performs reconstruction – the face, eyes, nose, ears, and breast.

He is currently the Director of the Microsurgery and Breast Fellowship, Director of the Facial Reanimation Program, Co-Director of the Adult Craniofacial Fellowship, Director of Clinical Research, and Director of the Medical Student Specialty rotation and courses.

Dr. Rozen is board-certified in plastic surgery and is a Diplomate of the American Board of Plastic Surgery and the American Board of Surgery, as well as a Fellow of the American College of Surgeons.

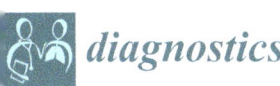

Editorial

Special Issue: Evidence-Based Diagnosis and Management of Facial Nerve Disorders

Gerd Fabian Volk [1,2,3,*], Caroline Cora Kraus [1,2], Steffen U. Eisenhardt [4] and Shai Rozen [5]

1. Department of Otorhinolaryngology, Jena University Hospital, Am Klinikum 1, 07747 Jena, Germany; caroline.cora.kraus@uni-jena.de
2. Facial-Nerve-Center Jena, Jena University Hospital, Am Klinikum 1, 07747 Jena, Germany
3. Center of Rare Diseases Jena, Jena University Hospital, Am Klinikum 1, 07747 Jena, Germany
4. Department of Plastic and Hand Surgery, Medical Center-University of Freiburg, Faculty of Medicine, University of Freiburg, 79106 Freiburg, Germany
5. University of Texas Southwestern Medical Center, Dallas, TX 75390, USA
* Correspondence: fabian.volk@med.uni-jena.de

Although there has been a rapid increase in the number of new publications and studies in relation to the diagnostics, impacts and rehabilitation methods of facial nerve disorders, a general structure in evidence-based medicine is still difficult to establish. With this Special Issue on the topic of "Evidence Based Diagnosis and Management of Facial Nerve Disorders", we brought together experts from various fields, including speech pathology, plastic surgery, otolaryngology, neurology, and physical therapy, to present the latest developments in relation to facial nerve disorders and to show a great variety of topics to our audience/readership.

There are a few case review studies on this fascinating condition, for example a retrospective examination from 1987 to 2018 on different variants of the treatment for facial nerve schwannoma and changes in facial nerve function afterwards [1], as well as a rare case of facial nerve palsy caused by "osteoradionecrosis of the temporal bone" [2], which is a "[...] rare, delayed complication after radiotherapy for head and neck cancer" [2].

Furthermore, the advance of different diagnostic methods and assessment is worthy of observation. The article by A. Kehrer et al., for example, attempts to "[...] outline the key steps in a [high-resolution ultrasound] examination and extract an optimized workflow schema" [3] in patients with post-palsy synkinesis, while other articles focus on electrodiagnostic methods with the aim of creating a more objective evaluation of nerve injuries [4], including the attempt to "[...] develop a standardized protocol for a reliable surface EMG examination of all nine ear muscles in twelve healthy participants" [5] which was then applied "[...] in seven patients with unilateral postparalytic facial synkinesis" [5]. Following that, we can also provide information about more recently developed methods, like the possibility of facial nerve palsy diagnostics via "[...] the use of regional information" [6] from photographs.

The impacts of facial nerve disorders on daily life, such as communication and also emotion recognition caused by different underlying conditions, are extremely relevant as well, and are intensively discussed in two articles which devote themselves to the subject of emotion recognition. The first one shows the testing of "[...] emotion recognition [...] in patients with central facial paresis after stroke" [7] in relation to a healthy control group, while the other one focuses on "[...] the effects of post-paralytic facial synkinesis on facial emotion recognition" [8].

Another aspect with utmost importance is the possibility of rehabilitation, which is outlined here in a conservative method described by C. E. Boschetti et al. in the form of a statistic comparison of patients participating or not participating in Kabat physical rehabilitation with "temporary facial nerve palsy after parotid tumor surgery" [9], while the article by H. Abing et al. evaluates an operative method by observing "[...] the time

Citation: Volk, G.F.; Kraus, C.C.; Eisenhardt, S.U.; Rozen, S. Special Issue: Evidence-Based Diagnosis and Management of Facial Nerve Disorders. *Diagnostics* **2023**, *13*, 3056. https://doi.org/10.3390/diagnostics13193056

Received: 9 August 2023
Accepted: 20 September 2023
Published: 26 September 2023

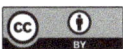

Copyright: © 2023 by the authors. Licensee MDPI, Basel, Switzerland. This article is an open access article distributed under the terms and conditions of the Creative Commons Attribution (CC BY) license (https://creativecommons.org/licenses/by/4.0/).

course of clinical and electromyographical (EMG) reinnervation after the reanimation of the smile using a gracilis muscle transplant which is reinnervated with the masseteric nerve" [10].

In conclusion, we can see that the topic of facial nerve palsy offers a vast and dynamic spectrum of developments in the fields of causation, diagnostics, and therapy/rehabilitation. We hope that the research presented in this Special Issue shows the importance of a multidisciplinary approach and will not only help to enhance our knowledge of this condition, but also ultimately improve patient outcomes and their quality of life.

Author Contributions: Writing—original draft preparation, C.C.K.; writing—review and editing, G.F.V., S.U.E. and S.R. All authors have read and agreed to the published version of the manuscript.

Conflicts of Interest: The author declares no conflict of interest.

References

1. Kitama, T.; Hosoya, M.; Noguchi, M.; Nishiyama, T.; Wakabayashi, T.; Shimanuki, M.N.; Yazawa, M.; Inoue, Y.; Kanzaki, J.; Ogawa, K.; et al. Intratemporal Facial Nerve Schwannomas: A Review of 45 Cases in A Single Center. *Diagnostics* **2022**, *12*, 1789. [CrossRef] [PubMed]
2. Schmidt, F.; Bradley, K.; Volk, G.F. Osteoradionecrosis of the Temporal Bone as a Rare Cause of Facial Nerve Palsy. *Diagnostics* **2022**, *12*, 1021. [CrossRef] [PubMed]
3. Kehrer, A.; Ruewe, M.; Platz Batista da Silva, N.; Lonic, D.; Heidekrueger, P.I.; Knoedler, S.; Jung, E.M.; Prantl, L.; Knoedler, L. Using High-Resolution Ultrasound to Assess Post-Facial Paralysis Synkinesis—Machine Settings and Technical Aspects for Facial Surgeons. *Diagnostics* **2022**, *12*, 1650. [CrossRef] [PubMed]
4. Yoo, M.C. Diagnostic Value of Preoperative Electrodiagnostic Analysis in a Patient with Facial Palsy and a Large Vestibular Schwannoma: Case Report. *Diagnostics* **2022**, *12*, 542. [CrossRef] [PubMed]
5. Rüschenschmidt, H.; Volk, G.F.; Anders, C.; Guntinas-Lichius, O. Electromyography of Extrinsic and Intrinsic Ear Muscles in Healthy Probands and Patients with Unilateral Postparalytic Facial Synkinesis. *Diagnostics* **2022**, *12*, 121. [CrossRef] [PubMed]
6. Parra-Dominguez, G.S.; Garcia-Capulin, C.H.; Sanchez-Yanez, R.E. Automatic Facial Palsy Diagnosis as a Classification Problem Using Regional Information Extracted from a Photograph. *Diagnostics* **2022**, *12*, 1528. [CrossRef] [PubMed]
7. Kuttenreich, A.-M.; von Piekartz, H.; Heim, S. Is There a Difference in Facial Emotion Recognition after Stroke with vs. without Cetral Facial Paresis? *Diagnostics* **2022**, *12*, 1721. [CrossRef] [PubMed]
8. Kuttenreich, A.-M.; Volk, G.F.; Guntinas-Lichius, O.; von Piekartz, H.; Heim, S. Facial Emotion Recognition in Patients with Post-Paralytic Facial Synkinesis—A Present Competence. *Diagnostics* **2022**, *12*, 1138. [CrossRef]
9. Boschetti, C.E.; Lo Giuidce, G.; Spuntarelli, C.; Apice, C.; Rauso, R.; Santagata, M.; Tartaro, G.; Colella, G. Kabat Rehabilitation in Facial Nerve Palsy after Parotid Gland Tumor Surgery: A Case-Control Study. *Diagnostics* **2022**, *12*, 565. [CrossRef]
10. Abing, H.; Pick, C.; Steffens, T.; Sharma, J.S.; Klußmann, J.P.; Grosheva, M. Reanimation of the Smile with Neuro-Vascular Anastomosed Gracilis Muscle: A Case Series. *Diagnostics* **2022**, *12*, 1282. [CrossRef] [PubMed]

Disclaimer/Publisher's Note: The statements, opinions and data contained in all publications are solely those of the individual author(s) and contributor(s) and not of MDPI and/or the editor(s). MDPI and/or the editor(s) disclaim responsibility for any injury to people or property resulting from any ideas, methods, instructions or products referred to in the content.

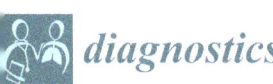

Article

Electromyography of Extrinsic and Intrinsic Ear Muscles in Healthy Probands and Patients with Unilateral Postparalytic Facial Synkinesis

Hanna Rüschenschmidt [1], Gerd Fabian Volk [1,2,3], Christoph Anders [4] and Orlando Guntinas-Lichius [1,2,3,*]

1. Department of Otorhinolaryngology, Jena University Hospital, 07747 Jena, Germany; hanna.rueschenschmidt@web.de (H.R.); fabian.volk@med.uni-jena.de (G.F.V.)
2. Facial Nerve Center, Jena University Hospital, 07747 Jena, Germany
3. Center for Rare Diseases, Jena University Hospital, 07747 Jena, Germany
4. Division for Motor Research, Pathophysiology and Biomechanics, Department for Trauma-, Hand- and Reconstructive Surgery, Jena University Hospital, 07743 Jena, Germany; christoph.anders@med.uni-jena.de
* Correspondence: orlando.guntinas@med.uni-jena.de; Tel.: +49-364-1932-9301; Fax: +49-364-1932-9302

Abstract: There are currently no data on the electromyography (EMG) of all intrinsic and extrinsic ear muscles. The aim of this work was to develop a standardized protocol for a reliable surface EMG examination of all nine ear muscles in twelve healthy participants. The protocol was then applied in seven patients with unilateral postparalytic facial synkinesis. Based on anatomic preparations of all ear muscles on two cadavers, hot spots for the needle EMG of each individual muscle were defined. Needle and surface EMG were performed in one healthy participant; facial movements could be defined for the reliable activation of individual ear muscles' surface EMG. In healthy participants, most tasks led to the activation of several ear muscles without any side difference. The greatest EMG activity was seen when smiling. Ipsilateral and contralateral gaze were the only movements resulting in very distinct activation of the transversus auriculae and obliquus auriculae muscles. In patients with facial synkinesis, ear muscles' EMG activation was stronger on the postparalytic compared to the contralateral side for most tasks. Additionally, synkinetic activation was verifiable in the ear muscles. The surface EMG of all ear muscles is reliably feasible during distinct facial tasks, and ear muscle EMG enriches facial electrodiagnostics.

Keywords: auricular muscles; facial muscles; human; facial palsy; electrophysiology; ear wiggling

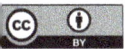

1. Introduction

The human auricle contains three extrinsic and six intrinsic muscles [1]. These muscles have been considered vestigial in humans, and are rarely under voluntary control [2]. Like the mimic muscles, all ear muscles are innervated by the facial nerve [1]. Needle and surface electromyography (EMG) are part of routine electrodiagnostics in patients with facial nerve dysfunction, mainly for facial palsy [3]. In these patients, EMG is routinely performed from the mimic muscles. EMG data on human ear muscles are sparse. Berzin and Fortinguerra published data for the three external muscles (anterior, superior and posterior auricular) of 30 healthy men [4]. They showed EMG activity in all these muscles but never isolated activity in only one muscle during smiling and yawning. Serra et al. analyzed the posterior auricular muscle in patients with acute facial paralysis [5]. Due to the acute paralysis, EMG activity disappears in this ear muscle like in mimic muscles. Posterior auricular muscle EMG activity preceded the recovery of EMG signs in other facial muscles by 10–30 days. Furthermore, they revealed in patients with postparalytic facial synkinesis synchronous EMG activity with the orbicularis oculi muscle during eye blink. This is a sign that the ear muscles are also involved in the process of postparalytic synkinesis. Recently, such postparalytic facial-auricular synkinesis was also reported in a case report [6]. The ear muscles are not only of interest in patients with facial palsy. The ear muscles are part of a complex neural brainstem network for the postauricular reflex [7]. Therefore, the measurement of ear muscle EMG activity offers so-far unexploited potential for the monitoring of emotional states, brainstem lesion diagnostics or stroke manifestations [2]. Finally, the ear muscles are beneficial for individuals with quadriplegia because these muscles are usually not affected by high-level spinal lesions [2]. For instance, such patients can learn to steer a wheelchair with ear muscle activation [8]. This also opens the field for other neuroprosthetic applications based on auricular muscles.

Therefore, we thought that it would be worthwhile to systematically investigate: (1) the exact localization of all extrinsic and intrinsic ear muscles in cadaver preparations for optimal placement of the EMG electrodes, (2) the EMG activity in all extrinsic and intrinsic ear muscles in healthy individuals and (3) the changes of EMG activity in patients with postparalytic facial synkinesis.

2. Material and Methods

This study was approved by the Ethics Committee of Jena University Hospital (No. 2018-1103-BO). All participants provided written informed consent. Twelve healthy probands (8 female, 4 male; age: 18–29 years) were examined by one-channel and multi-channel EMG. Additionally, needle EMG was performed in one healthy proband only. Surface EMG was performed in all 12 probands. Seven patients (4 female, 3 male; age: 18–60 years) with postparalytic facial synkinesis after acute unilateral (5 right side, 2 left side) peripheral facial paralysis (mean time since onset: 34.7 months) were examined. The patients received surface one-channel EMG. All measurements were performed on both sides of the face. Additionally, the anatomical preparations were performed on two hemifaces.

2.1. Cadaver Preparations

First, cadaver preparations were performed to better understand the exact localization and size of the ear muscles. The anatomical preparations were carried out on two hemifaces from body donors at the forensic medicine department of the University Hospital Hamburg-Eppendorf, Germany. First, the pre-, supra- and postauricular cutis and subcutis were dissected. The scalp was detached from ventral to dorsal around the cartilaginous auricle. As the auricular muscles are not different to other facial muscles, they were not covered by fascia. After removing the subcutaneous fat tissue, the three extrinsic ear muscles could be visualized. For the preparation of the ventral side of the auricle, the cutis was dissected away from the cartilage and the cartilaginous tragus exposed. For further dissection of the tragicus muscle, the cartilage was slit on the dorsal posterior margin of the tragus so that the cartilage could be unfolded. The helicis major and helicis minor muscles were exposed on the crus helicis. Following the course of the helix, the skin was detached down to the earlobe and the antitragicus muscle was exposed. Finally, the transversus auriculae and the obliquus auriculae muscle were dissected on the back side after removal of the cutis.

The photographic documentation of the prepared ear muscles was compared with anatomical drawings from anatomy atlases [1,9–12]. Both were used as a guide for the positioning of the fine needle electrodes and surface electrodes. Graphics were created which illustrate the size and position of the ear muscles and on which the exact positioning of the electrodes could be displayed.

2.2. One-Channel Needle and Surface Electromyography Setting

Needle EMGs were first performed in one healthy proband using optimal recording spots based on the cadaver dissections. The region of optimal signaling was thereafter used for the surface EMG recordings. A standard EMG system was used (Medelec Synergy T5, VIASYS Healthcare, Höchberg, Germany; high-pass filter: 20 Hz; low-pass filter: 5 kHz). For needle EMG, concentric electrodes were used (Neuroline concentric needle, 50 × 0.45 mm; Ambu, Bad Nauheim, Germany). For surface EMG, surface electrodes were applied (Neuroline 720 Neurology Surface Electrodes 72015- K/10, Ambu, Bad Nauheim, Germany).

All EMG examinations were performed in supine position. The auricle and surrounding skin were disinfected and degreased with a skin disinfectant. The reference electrode was positioned on the spinous process of the seventh cervical vertebra. Only before performing the needle EMGs were the puncture sites anesthetized with an anesthetic cream (EMLA; 25 mg/g lidocaine plus 25 mg/g prilocaine, Aspen, Munich, Germany). In healthy probands, the examinations started on the left side, followed by the right side. In patients, first the contralateral side and then the affected sided was analyzed. The sequence of recordings was always the same: auricularis anterior, auricularis superior, auricularis posterior, tragicus, antitragicus, helicis major, helicis minor, transversus auriculae and finally obliquus auriculae muscle. The probands had to perform the following mimic exercises, always in the same sequence: smiling, pursing lips, nose wrinkling, frowning, drawing eyebrows together, ipsilateral gaze, contralateral gaze and finally ear wiggling. Each task was performed 48 times. The movements were demonstrated by the examiner and practiced together with the examiner before starting the recordings. For quality control, all EMG recordings were video-documented (Supplementary Figure S1). The amplitude of the EMG signal from the recorded ear muscle during the specific exercise was evaluated off-line using the video recordings and the following standard 4-point classification system [3]: no increase compared to baseline activity in resting state (=0), slight increase (=1), moderate increase (=2) and strong increase (=3). Examples for the classification are shown in Supplementary Figure S1.

2.3. Multi-Channel Surface Electromyography Setting

For multi-channel EMG, a standard EMG system (Tower of Measurement, DeMeTec, Langgöns, Germany) and amplifier (Biovision, Wehrheim, Germany; sampling rate: 4096 Hz; amplitude resolution: 60 nV/bit) were used. Three ear muscles (auricularis superior, auricularis posterior, tragicus), a mimic muscle (risorius) and two chewing muscles (temporalis, masseter) were synchronously recorded. The recordings were performed in a sitting position. Surface electrodes (Kendall EGC electrodes H93SG, 42 mm × 24 mm; Covidien, Dublin, Ireland) were applied (Supplementary Figure S2). These electrodes have the advantage that they can be trimmed. By trimming, electrode overlap can be avoided. The probands had to perform the following mimic exercises, always in the same sequence as described for the single-channel recording (see above). In addition, the following tasks were performed: showing teeth, clenching teeth, chewing on the ipsilateral side and chewing on the contralateral side. All EMG recordings were video-documented. For classification of the EMG activity, the same classification systems as for the single-channel analysis were used (see above).

2.4. Statistical Analysis

Statistical analyses were performed using Microsoft Excel (V.2016, Microsoft Corporation, Seattle, WA, USA) and using IBM SPSS v.26.0 statistical software for Windows (Chicago, IL, USA). If not otherwise reported, mean values ± standard deviations of the EMG recordings of the healthy probands or the patients are presented. Differences between two dependent subgroups (right versus left side in healthy probands or postparalytic side versus contralateral side) for ordinal EMG classification data were compared with the Wilcoxon test. For all statistical tests, significance was two-sided and set to $p < 0.05$.

3. Results
3.1. Cadaver Preparations of the Extrinsic and Intrinsic Ear Muscles

Supplementary Figure S3 summarizes the preparations of the ear muscles. Nearly all muscles could be detected. The helicis minor muscle could not be clearly depicted in both cadavers. The tragicus and the antitragicus were located within the tragal and antitragal cartilage, respectively. The auricularis posterior muscle had two muscle bellies in one cadaver. The transversus auriculae muscle was clearly visible in only one preparation. Optimal spots for the surface EMG recordings of all ear muscles (Figure 1) were defined based on the cadaver preparations and needle EMG results (see below).

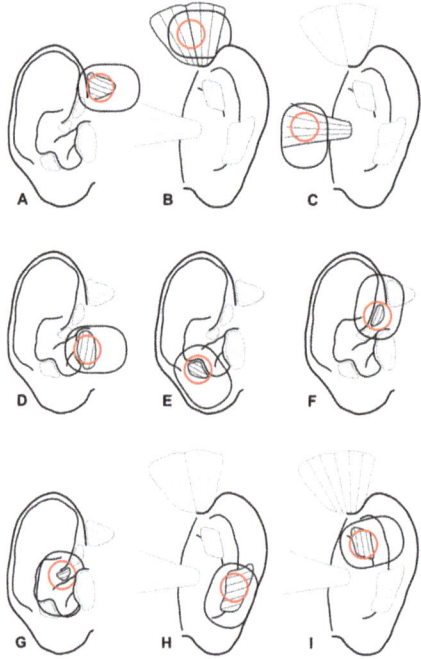

Figure 1. Localization of the extrinsic and intrinsic ear muscles for EMG analysis. (**A**): M. auricularis anterior. (**B**): M. auricularis superior. (**C**): M. auricularis posterior. (**D**): M. tragicus. (**E**): M. antitragicus. (**F**): M. helicis major. (**G**): M. helicis minor. (**H**): M. obliquus auriculae. (**I**): M. transversus auriculae.

3.2. One-Channel Needle Electromyography of the Extrinsic and Intrinsic Ear Muscles in One Healthy Proband

Except for the transversus auriculae muscle on the left side and the obliquus auriculae muscle on the right side, needle EMG was feasible for all extrinsic and intrinsic ear muscles (Supplementary Table S1). The optimal hot spots for the needle EMG of individual ear muscles are shown in Supplementary Figure S4. Overall, the external muscles showed higher activity than the intrinsic muscles. The strongest activity was seen in all muscles during ear wiggling and smiling. The obliquus auriculae showed the weakest activity. The transversus auriculae was only activated during lateral gaze. Frowning only activated the extrinsic ear muscles, whereas the same muscles showed no activity during drawing of the eyebrows together. The activity pattern during needle EMG was not significantly different from surface EMG in the one individual receiving both needle and surface EMG analyses (data of the comparison not shown).

3.3. One-Channel Surface Electromyography of the Extrinsic and Intrinsic Ear Muscles in Healthy Probands

Surface EMG could be recorded from all ear muscles in all healthy subjects. There was no significant right–left side difference (Table 1). In general, the ear muscle EMG activity was highest during smiling and ear wiggling. The lowest activity was seen during ipsilateral or contralateral gaze. Only the obliquus auriculae and the transversus auriculae muscle showed a robust activity during the isolated lateral gaze.

Table 1. Healthy probands: average surface single-channel EMG activity * in the different ear muscles during mimic tasks on right and left sides.

Muscle/Exercise	Right Side	Left Side	p	Muscle/Exercise	Right Side	Left Side	p	Muscle/Exercise	Right Side	Left Side	p
M. auricularis ant.	Mean ± SD	Mean ± SD		M. tragicus	Mean ± SD	Mean ± SD		M. helicis minor	Mean ± SD	Mean ± SD	
Smiling	2.91 ± 0.28	2.83 ± 0.38	0.586	Smiling	2.90 ± 0.30	3.00 ± 0	0.341	Smiling	2.77 ± 0.44	2.77 ± 0.44	1.000
Pursing lips	1.41 ± 0.79	1.66 ± 0.88	0.339	Pursing lips	1.54 ± 0.82	1.81 ± 0.60	0.277	Pursing lips	1.00 ± 1.11	1.44 ± 1.01	0.272
Nose wrinkling	0.66 ± 0.65	1.41 ± 1.08	0.069	Nose wrinkling	0.90 ± 0.87	0.80 ± 0.78	0.780	Nose wrinkling	0.11 ± 0.33	0.77 ± 1.09	0.050
Frowning	1.91 ± 1.16	1.33 ± 1.15	0.189	Frowning	1 ± 0.89	1.45 ± 1.03	0.096	Frowning	1.55 ± 1.33	1.33 ± 1.41	0.347
Drawing eyebrows	0.33 ± 0.88	0.58 ± 0.66	0.491	Drawing eyebrows	0.18 ± 0.60	0.90 ± 0.94	0.054	Drawing eyebrows	0.11 ± 0.33	0.44 ± 1.01	0.347
Ipsilateral gaze	0.41 ± 0.90	0.58 ± 0.79	0.504	Ipsilateral gaze	0.27 ± 0.90	0.18 ± 0.4	0.779	Ipsilateral gaze	0 ± 0	0.33 ± 0.70	0.195
Contralateral gaze	0	0.45 ± 0.52	0.016	Contralateral gaze	0.18 ± 0.60	0.27 ± 0.64	0.756	Contralateral gaze	0.22 ± 0.44	0.22 ± 0.44	1.000
Ear wiggling	2.75 ± 0.7	2.75 ± 0.7	NA	Ear wiggling	2.42 ± 0.78	2.42 ± 0.97	1.000	Ear wiggling	2.83 ± 0.4	2.5 ± 1.22	0.363
M. auricularis sup.				M. antitragicus				M. trans. auriculae			
Smiling	2.83 ± 0.38	2.83 ± 0.38	1.000	Smiling	2.91 ± 0.28	2.83 ± 0.57	0.339	Smiling	3 ± 0	2.91 ± 0.28	0.339
Pursing lips	1.16 ± 1.02	1.41 ± 0.9	0.339	Pursing lips	1.41 ± 0.79	1.33 ± 0.98	0.795	Pursing lips	1.16 ± 0.83	1.16 ± 0.71	1.000
Nose wrinkling	0.91 ± 1.08	0.66 ± 0.77	0.389	Nose wrinkling	0.58 ± 0.79	0.58 ± 0.79	1.000	Nose wrinkling	0.66 ± 0.88	1.08 ± 0.90	0.137
Frowning	2.25 ± 0.96	2.25 ± 0.96	1.000	Frowning	1.45 ± 1.21	1.54 ± 1.21	0.756	Frowning	1.66 ± 1.30	1.50 ± 1.24	0.504
Drawing eyebrows	0.50 ± 0.90	0.75 ± 0.96	0.191	Drawing eyebrows	0.33 ± 0.77	1.00 ± 1.04	0.071	Drawing eyebrows	0.50 ± 1.00	0.41 ± 0.66	0.586
Ipsilateral gaze	0.83 ± 1.19	1.00 ± 0.85	0.674	Ipsilateral gaze	0.50 ± 0.90	0.25 ± 0.45	0.339	Ipsilateral gaze	1.16 ± 1.11	1.00 ± 0.85	0.615
Contralateral gaze	0.25 ± 0.62	0.33 ± 0.65	0.723	Contralateral gaze	0.66 ± 0.77	0.33 ± 0.49	0.220	Contralateral gaze	1.25 ± 0.96	1.00 ± 0.95	0.463
Ear wiggling	2.87 ± 0.35	2.75 ± 0.46	0.351	Ear wiggling	2.85 ± 0.37	2.57 ± 1.13	0.356	Ear wiggling	2.75 ± 0.46	2.50 ± 0.92	0.170
M. auricularis post.				M. helicis major				M. obliq. auriculae			
Smiling	2.41 ± 0.51	2.58 ± 0.66	0.339	Smiling	3.00 ± 0	2.81 ± 0.4	0.167	Smiling	2.90 ± 0.30	3 ± 0	0.341
Pursing lips	0.91 ± 0.9	1.16 ± 0.93	0.389	Pursing lips	1.18 ± 0.98	0.9 ± 1.13	0.465	Pursing lips	1.00 ± 0.89	1.18 ± 0.98	0.506
Nose wrinkling	0.58 ± 0.79	0.75 ± 0.75	0.551	Nose wrinkling	1.18 ± 1.25	0.9 ± 0.83	0.341	Nose wrinkling	0.72 ± 1.00	0.90 ± 1.04	0.441
Frowning	1.41 ± 1.44	1.83 ± 1.46	0.210	Frowning	2.45 ± 0.93	1.9 ± 1.04	0.052	Frowning	1.90 ± 1.22	1.90 ± 1.22	1.000
Drawing eyebrows	0.50 ± 0.90	0.83 ± 1.19	0.266	Drawing eyebrows	0.63 ± 0.92	0.72 ± 1.00	0.810	Drawing eyebrows	0.90 ± 1.13	0.63 ± 0.80	0.082
Ipsilateral gaze	1.00 ± 0.95	0.83 ± 0.57	0.586	Ipsilateral gaze	0.36 ± 0.8	0.36 ± 0.5	1.000	Ipsilateral gaze	1.27 ± 0.90	1.00 ± 0.89	0.432
Contralateral gaze	0.66 ± 1.07	0.75 ± 0.75	0.809	Contralateral gaze	0.18 ± 0.4	0.18 ± 0.4	1.000	Contralateral gaze	1.18 ± 0.98	1.27 ± 1.10	0.821
Ear wiggling	2.62 ± 0.74	2.75 ± 0.46	0.351	Ear wiggling	2.86 ± 0.37	2.86 ± 0.37	NA	Ear wiggling	2.87 ± 0.35	2.50 ± 0.92	0.197

* EMG classification: 0 = no increase compared to baseline activity in resting state, 1 = slight increase, 2 = moderate increase, 3 = strong increase.

3.4. Multi-Channel Surface Electromyography of the Extrinsic and Intrinsic Ear Muscles in Healthy Probands

The mimic exercises (smiling, pursing lips, nose wrinkling, frowning, drawing eyebrows together, showing teeth) activated the risorius as a mimic muscle, but also synchronously at least two ear muscles and one or both chewing muscles (Table 2). Ear wiggling showed the strongest co-activation of all recorded muscles. The co-activation during the lateral gaze was weaker but clearly visible in mimic and ear muscles, but very weak in the temporalis muscle. The masseter showed no activity during the lateral gaze movements. The chewing tasks (clenching teeth, chewing ipsilateral, chewing contralateral) triggered a strong activation in all muscles except for the auricularis posterior muscles. This muscle remained silent during chewing tasks.

Table 2. Healthy probands: average surface multi-channel EMG activity * synchronously in several ear muscles, chewing muscles and one mimic muscle during different tasks summarized for both sided of the face.

Exercise	M. risorius	M. auricularis Posterior	M. auricularis Superior	M. tragicus	M. temporalis	M. masseter
	Mean ± SD	Mean ± SD	Mean ± SD	Mean ± SD	Mean ± SD	Mean ± SD
Smiling	2.64 + 0.50	0 + 0	2.64 + 0.50	1.91 + 1.51	2.00 + 0	1.64 + 0.50
Pursing lips	2.27 + 1.01	0 + 0	1.91 + 0.30	0.64 + 0.50	1.82 + 0.40	0.64 + 0.50
Nose wrinkling	1.09 + 0.30	0 + 0	1.36 + 0.50	0.64 + 0.50	1.00 + 0	0 + 0
Frowning	1.64 + 0.50	1.36 + 0.50	2.91 + 0.30	1.36 + 0.50	3.00 + 0	1.00 + 0
Drawing eyebrows	2.36 + 0.50	0.36 + 0.50	2 + 0	1.09 + 1.51	2.36 + 0.50	1.00 + 0
Ipsilateral gaze	1.82 + 0.98	0 + 0	1.64 + 0.50	0.36 + 0.50	1.73 + 1.01	1.09 + 1.51
Contralateral gaze	1.64 + 0.92	0 + 0	2.36 + 0.50	1.00 + 1.41	1.73 + 1.01	1.09 + 1.51
Ear wiggling	1.64 + 0.92	1.27 + 1.01	3.00 + 0	2.27 + 0.47	3.00 + 0	1.64 + 0.92
Showing teeth	3.00 + 0	0.64 + 0.50	2.27 + 0.47	3.00 + 0	2.64 + 0.50	1.36 + 0.50
Clenching teeth	3.00 + 0	0 + 0	1.36 + 0.50	1.09 + 0.30	2.64 + 0.50	2.27 + 1.01
Chewing ipsilateral	2.27 + 1.01	0 + 0	2.18 + 0.98	2.09 + 0.94	2.18 + 0.98	1.73 + 1.42
Chewing contralateral	2.55 + 0.52	0.36 + 0.50	3.00 + 0	2.27 + 1.01	2.91 + 0.3	2.27 + 1.01

* EMG classification: 0 = no increase compared to baseline activity in resting state, 1 = slight increase, 2 = moderate increase, 3 = strong increase.

3.5. One-Channel Surface Electromyography of the Extrinsic and Intrinsic Ear Muscles in Patients with Postparalytic Facial Synkinesis

Like in healthy individuals, the strongest EMG activity in ear muscles was seen during smiling on both sides, and for ear wiggling on the contralateral side (Table 3). Interestingly, the activity on the postparalytic side was much lower during ear wiggling. Especially, nose wrinkling showed a much higher activity on the postparalytic side than in normal individuals. The average EMG activity was always higher on the postparalytic side than on the contralateral side. An example for the anterior and posterior muscles is shown in Figure 2. Even in this small sample size, the difference was significantly different ($p < 0.05$) for several muscles and tasks. EMG activity was also seen in other ear muscles than the obliquus auriculae and the transversus auriculae muscle.

Table 3. Patients with postparalytic facial synkinesis: average surface single-channel EMG activity * in the different ear muscles during mimic tasks on postparalytic and contralateral sides.

Muscle/Exercise	Postparalytic	Contralateral	p	Muscle/Exercise	Postparalytic	Contralateral	p	Muscle/Exercise	Postparalytic	Contralateral	p
M. auricularis ant.	Mean ± SD	Mean ± SD		M. tragicus	Mean ± SD	Mean ± SD		M. helicis minor	Mean ± SD	Mean ± SD	
Smiling	2.71 ± 0.48	2.85 ± 0.37	0.356	Smiling	2.28 ± 0.75	2.71 ± 0.48	0.078	Smiling	2.85 ± 0.37	2.57 ± 0.53	0.172
Pursing lips	1.71 ± 1.25	1.00 ± 0.57	0.140	Pursing lips	1.57 ± 0.78	0.71 ± 0.48	0.001	Pursing lips	1.85 ± 1.06	0.57 ± 0.53	0.012
Nose wrinkling	2 ± 1	1.28 ± 1.25	0.310	Nose wrinkling	1.71 ± 0.75	1.00 ± 1.00	0.094	Nose wrinkling	2 ± 0.57	0.71 ± 0.95	0.022
Frowning	2.28 ± 0.75	1.85 ± 0.89	0.356	Frowning	2 ± 0.81	1.42 ± 0.97	0.280	Frowning	2.14 ± 0.69	1.28 ± 0.75	0.078
Drawing eyebrows	1.85 ± 1.21	0.42 ± 0.53	0.016	Drawing eyebrows	1.71 ± 0.48	0.85 ± 0.89	0.045	Drawing eyebrows	1.85 ± 0.89	0.14 ± 0.37	0.007
Ipsilateral gaze	1.28 ± 0.75	0.42 ± 0.53	0.078	Ipsilateral gaze	0.42 ± 0.53	1.00 ± 1.15	0.103	Ipsilateral gaze	1.14 ± 0.89	0.28 ± 0.48	0.045
Contralateral gaze	0.42 ± 0.78	0.57 ± 0.78	0.604	Contralateral gaze	0.42 ± 0.53	0.71 ± 1.11	0.604	Contralateral gaze	0.28 ± 0.48	0.42 ± 0.53	0.604
Ear wiggling	1.33 ± 1.15	2.66 ± 0.57	0.270	Ear wiggling	1.33 ± 1.52	2.33 ± 0.57	0.225	Ear wiggling	1.33 ± 1.52	2.66 ± 0.57	0.184
M auricularis sup.				M. antitragicus				M. trans. auriculae			
Smiling	2.57 ± 0.78	2.85 ± 0.37	0.356	Smiling	2.42 ± 0.53	2.71 ± 0.48	0.172	Smiling	2.71 ± 0.48	2.57 ± 0.53	0.356
Pursing lips	2.28 ± 1.11	1.28 ± 0.75	0.018	Pursing lips	1.85 ± 1.06	0.57 ± 0.78	0.035	Pursing lips	1.85 ± 0.69	1.00 ± 0.81	0.078

Table 3. *Cont.*

Muscle/Exercise	Postparalytic	Contralateral	p	Muscle/Exercise	Postparalytic	Contralateral	p	Muscle/Exercise	Postparalytic	Contralateral	p
Nose wrinkling	2.28 ± 0.75	1.00 ± 1.15	0.093	Nose wrinkling	2.28 ± 0.75	0.57 ± 1.13	**0.011**	Nose wrinkling	2.42 ± 0.53	1.14 ± 1.06	0.063
Frowning	2.28 ± 0.75	1.85 ± 1.06	0.510	Frowning	2 ± 0.81	1.14 ± 0.37	**0.017**	Frowning	1.71 ± 0.95	1.42 ± 0.53	0.522
Drawing eyebrows	2.28 ± 1.11	0.42 ± 0.53	**0.004**	Drawing eyebrows	1.28 ± 1.25	0.28 ± 0.75	**0.038**	Drawing eyebrows	1.71 ± 0.75	0.71 ± 0.95	0.062
Ipsilateral gaze	1.28 ± 1.11	1.00 ± 1.00	0.457	Ipsilateral gaze	1 ± 0.57	0.57 ± 0.53	0.078	Ipsilateral gaze	0.85 ± 0.69	1.28 ± 0.95	0.289
Contralateral gaze	0.85 ± 1.21	0.71 ± 0.75	0.766	Contralateral gaze	0.42 ± 0.53	0.42 ± 0.78	1.000	Contralateral gaze	0.57 ± 0.53	1.42 ± 1.13	0.111
Ear wiggling	2 ± 1	2.33 ± 0.57	0.742	Ear wiggling	1 ± 1.73	2.00 ± 1.00	0.225	Ear wiggling	1.33 ± 1.52	2.00 ± 1.00	0.667
M. auricularis post.				**M. helicis major**				**M. obliq. auriculae**			
Smiling	2.71 ± 0.48	2.28 ± 0.48	0.200	Smiling	3 ± 0	3.00 ± 0	NA	Smiling	2.71 ± 0.48	2.57 ± 0.53	0.356
Pursing lips	1.85 ± 0.89	0.71 ± 0.75	**0.005**	Pursing lips	1.71 ± 1.11	0.57 ± 0.53	**0.047**	Pursing lips	1.85 ± 1.06	0.71 ± 0.95	0.103
Nose wrinkling	2.57 ± 0.53	1.14 ± 1.21	**0.008**	Nose wrinkling	2.42 ± 0.53	1.42 ± 1.13	0.086	Nose wrinkling	2.28 ± 0.48	1.14 ± 1.21	0.066
Frowning	2.14 ± 0.69	1.57 ± 1.27	0.413	Frowning	2.57 ± 0.53	1.71 ± 0.95	**0.017**	Frowning	2 ± 1	1.85 ± 0.89	0.604
Drawing eyebrows	2 ± 1.15	0.28 ± 0.48	**0.007**	Drawing eyebrows	2.14 ± 0.69	0.28 ± 0.75	**0.0001**	Drawing eyebrows	1.71 ± 0.75	0.43 ± 0.54	**0.022**
Ipsilateral gaze	1.14 ± 1.06	1.00 ± 0.81	0.736	Ipsilateral gaze	0.85 ± 0.69	0.28 ± 0.48	**0.030**	Ipsilateral gaze	0.71 ± 0.48	1.28 ± 1.11	0.231
Contralateral gaze	0.85 ± 0.69	1.00 ± 0.81	0.604	Contralateral gaze	0.42 ± 0.53	0.42 ± 0.53	1.000	Contralateral gaze	0.71 ± 0.48	1.71 ± 1.25	0.111
Ear wiggling	2 ± 1	2.66 ± 0.57	0.423	Ear wiggling	1.33 ± 1.52	2.33 ± 1.15	0.225	Ear wiggling	1.33 ± 1.52	2.66 ± 0.57	0.184

* EMG classification: 0 = no increase compared to baseline activity in resting state, 1 = slight increase, 2 = moderate increase, 3 = strong increase; significant values ($p < 0.05$) in bold.

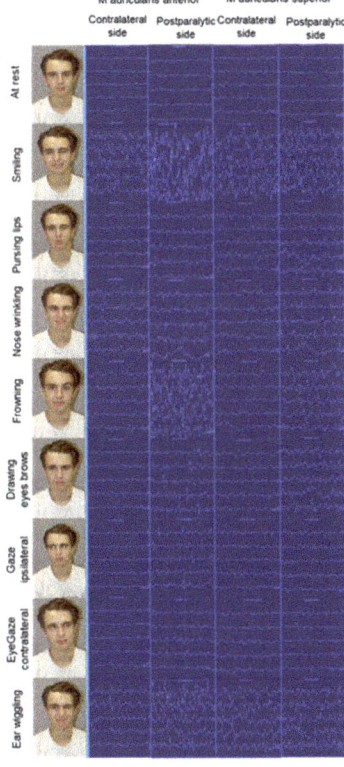

Figure 2. Example of a patient with postparalytic facial synkinesis on the left side. For most mimic tasks, the single-channel EMG activity was heavily increased on the postparalytic side in comparison to the contralateral side, here shown for the auricularis anterior and superior muscles.

4. Discussion

With this work, data are available for the first time on the implementation of EMGs on all intrinsic and extrinsic ear muscles. The co-activation of the ear muscles when smiling, pursing the lips, wrinkling the nose and making other facial movements could be shown by means of surface and needle EMG recordings. The results of the needle EMG with its very high spatial resolution and a measuring field of only approximately one cubic millimeter were important to define the hot spots for the recording and to confirm that the measured activity actually came from the inserted ear muscles of interest and not from the much larger neighboring muscles (e.g., the masseter muscles). Surface EMGs of all extrinsic and intrinsic ear muscles were feasible and meaningful, since individual activity patterns could be determined during co-activation through facial movements. Synchronous activation of ear muscles was the rule, and isolated activation was the exception. Hence, the results of Berzin and Fortinguerra could be confirmed for all ear muscles [4].

The postauricular muscle reflex activates the posterior auricular muscle in response to short and abrupt sounds [13]. This brainstem reflex is of interest because it is preserved in case of facial nerve lesion distal to the stylomastoid foramen but disturbed after more proximal lesions [14]. This reflex was not measured in the current study, but should be included in future investigations. However, the oculo-auricular phenomenon (i.e., the co-activation of ear muscles during lateral gaze) was investigated [15]. In concordance with previous investigations, we could show that especially ipsilateral gaze led to a strong (sometimes isolated) activation of the transversus auriculae and obliquus auriculae muscles [15]. Furthermore, it could be confirmed that lateral gaze enhances postauricular muscle reflex [16].

Needle electromyography is the standard method to objectively confirm facial synkinesis—that is, the abnormal involuntary facial movement that occurs with voluntary movement of a different facial muscle group [3]. Surface EMG also makes it possible to prove facial synkinesis [17]. The present study is the first to systematically show that postparalytic synkinesis also includes the extrinsic and intrinsic ear muscles. We showed complex patterns of involuntary ear muscle activity during mimic tasks beyond the typical synkinesis patterns seen in the mimic muscles of the patients. In most cases the EMG activity was heavily increased in comparison to the activity normally seen in these small muscles. One case report was published in 2020 showing oculo-auricular or oro-auricular synkinesis during similar mimic tasks, as in the present study [6]. Analysis of the ear muscles should be included into the repertoire of facial-muscle EMG analysis for patients with facial nerve diseases. Most ear muscles are innervated by the posterior auricular nerve [18]. Only the superior and anterior auricular muscles are innervated by the temporal branches of the facial nerve. The posterior auricular nerve arises from the facial nerve close to the stylomastoid foramen. Therefore, ear muscle EMG should be helpful to differentiate between intratemporal and extratemporal facial nerve trauma.

The study had several limitations. A standard examination procedure could be established and the ear muscle EMGs were highly reproducible, but overall the sample sizes of healthy volunteers and patients with postparalytic facial synkinesis were low. During most tasks, the average EMG activation was higher on the postparalytic than on the contralateral side. Due to the small samples, the difference reached a statistically significant difference only for some of these results. We expect clearer results when increasing the sample sizes in the future. The qualitative score to assess the changes in EMG activity was derived from clinical EMG scores used for the classification of facial muscle EMG [3]. Schmidt and Thoden use a similar score for classifying ear muscle activity [19]. To check the reproducibility of the evaluation of the EMGs by means of the qualitative score, an evaluation of the EMG activity changes by different examiners will be necessary in future trials. Even better, an automated EMG analysis should be developed. Recently, such a system was developed for the automated analysis of multi-channel mimic muscle EMG recordings [20].

Another recent study demonstrated that the ability to activate the posterior auricular muscle can be learned and used intuitively to steer a wheelchair with a myoelectric auricular control system [8]. The present study also shows that the other ear muscles show sufficient and reproducible activity to be used by assistive technologies even for more complex steering or other tasks.

5. Conclusions

Surface EMG recordings of all intrinsic and extrinsic ear muscles were feasible and reproducible. Distinct mimic movement tasks in which the ear muscles are active were defined. Mostly, several ear muscles were activated. Furthermore, in patients with postparalytic facial nerve syndrome, synkinetic activation of the ear muscles is the rule.

Supplementary Materials: The following supporting information can be downloaded at: https://www.mdpi.com/article/10.3390/diagnostics12010121/s1, Figure S1: Classification system for the EMG activity during the mimic tasks.; Figure S2: Example for the setting of the single-channel EMG recording with a patient in supine position on the left side and for multi-channel surface EMG recordings on the right side.; Figure S3: Cadaver preparations of the ear muscles.; Figure S4: Hot spots for needle EMG for each individual ear muscle shown on the left ear.; Table S1: Needle single-channel EMG activity* in the different ear muscles during mimic tasks on right and left side in one healthy probands.

Author Contributions: Conceptualization, O.G.-L., G.F.V. and C.A.; methodology, O.G.-L., G.F.V. and C.A.; formal analysis, H.R. and O.G.-L.; investigation, H.R.; resources, O.G.-L. and C.A.; writing—original draft preparation, O.G.-L.; writing—review and editing, all authors; visualization, H.R. and O.G.-L. All authors have read and agreed to the published version of the manuscript.

Funding: The study was sponsored by MED-EL Elektromedizinische Geräte GmbH, Innsbruck, Austria. Orlando Guntinas-Lichius acknowledges support by a Deutsche Forschungsgemeinschaft (DFG) grant GU-463/12-1.

Institutional Review Board Statement: The study was conducted in accordance with the Declaration of Helsinki, and approved by the Ethics Committee of Jena University Hospital, Jena, Germany (protocol code No. 2018-1103-BO, April 2018).

Informed Consent Statement: Informed consent was obtained from all subjects involved in the study.

Data Availability Statement: The datasets used during the current study are available from the corresponding author upon request.

Conflicts of Interest: The authors declare no conflict of interest.

References

1. Paulsen, F.; Waschke, J. *Atlas of Anatomy. Head, Neck and Neuroanatomy*; Elsevier: Amsterdam, The Netherlands, 2017; Volume 3.
2. Liugan, M.; Zhang, M.; Cakmak, Y.O. Neuroprosthetics for Auricular Muscles: Neural Networks and Clinical Aspects. *Front. Neurol.* **2017**, *8*, 752. [CrossRef] [PubMed]
3. Guntinas-Lichius, O.; Volk, G.F.; Olsen, K.D.; Makitie, A.A.; Silver, C.E.; Zafereo, M.E.; Rinaldo, A.; Randolph, G.W.; Simo, R.; Shaha, A.R.; et al. Facial nerve electrodiagnostics for patients with facial palsy: A clinical practice guideline. *Eur. Arch. Otorhinolaryngol.* **2020**, *277*, 1855–1874. [CrossRef] [PubMed]
4. Berzin, F.; Fortinguerra, C.R. EMG study of the anterior, superior and posterior auricular muscles in man. *Ann. Anat.* **1993**, *175*, 195–197. [CrossRef]
5. Serra, G.; Tugnoli, V.; Cristofori, M.C.; Eleopra, R.; de Grandis, D. The electromyographic examination of the posterior auricular muscle. *Electromyogr. Clin. Neurophysiol.* **1986**, *26*, 661–665. [PubMed]
6. Hobson, D.E.; Borys, A.E. Oculo-Auricular Synkinesia Post Bell's Palsy Causing Unilateral Wilson's Phenomenon. *Mov. Disord. Clin. Pract.* **2020**, *7*, 564–566. [CrossRef] [PubMed]
7. O'Beirne, G.A.; Patuzzi, R.B. Basic properties of the sound-evoked post-auricular muscle response (PAMR). *Hear. Res.* **1999**, *138*, 115–132. [CrossRef]
8. Schmalfuss, L.; Rupp, R.; Tuga, M.R.; Kogut, A.; Hewitt, M.; Meincke, J.; Klinker, F.; Duttenhoefer, W.; Eck, U.; Mikut, R.; et al. Steer by ear: Myoelectric auricular control of powered wheelchairs for individuals with spinal cord injury. *Restor. Neurol. Neurosci.* **2016**, *34*, 79–95. [CrossRef] [PubMed]
9. Kopsch, F. *Rauber's Lehrbuch der Anatomie des Menschen*, 8th ed.; Georg Thieme: Leipzig, Germany, 1909.
10. Platzer, W. *Pernkopf Anatomie: Kopf und Hals*; Urban & Schwarzenberg: Munich, Germany, 1987; Volume 1.

11. Benninghoff, A.; Drenckhahn, D. *Anatomie*; Elsevier: Amsterdam, The Netherlands, 2008.
12. Standring, S. *Gray's Anatomy. The Anatomical Basis of Clinical Practice*, 42nd ed.; Elsevier: Amsterdam, The Netherlands, 2020.
13. Benning, S.D.; Patrick, C.J.; Lang, A.R. Emotional modulation of the post-auricular reflex. *Psychophysiology* **2004**, *41*, 426–432. [CrossRef] [PubMed]
14. Bochenek, W.; Bochenek, Z. Postauricular (12 msec latency) responses to acoustic stimuli in patients with peripheral, facial nerve palsy. *Acta Otolaryngol.* **1976**, *81*, 264–269. [CrossRef] [PubMed]
15. Urban, P.P.; Marczynski, U.; Hopf, H.C. The oculo-auricular phenomenon. Findings in normals and patients with brainstem lesions. *Brain* **1993**, *116*, 727–738. [CrossRef] [PubMed]
16. Cook, A.; Patuzzi, R. Rotation of the eyes (not the head) potentiates the postauricular muscle response. *Ear Hear.* **2014**, *35*, 230–235. [CrossRef] [PubMed]
17. Bernardes, D.F.F.; Bento, R.F.; Goffi Gomez, M.V.S. The Contribution of Surface Electromyographic Assessment for Defining the Stage of Peripheral Facial Paralysis: Flaccid or Sequelae Stage. *Int. Arch. Otorhinolaryngol.* **2018**, *22*, 348–357. [CrossRef] [PubMed]
18. Smith, O.J.; Ross, G.L. Variations in the anatomy of the posterior auricular nerve and its potential as a landmark for identification of the facial nerve trunk: A cadaveric study. *Anat. Sci. Int.* **2012**, *87*, 101–105. [CrossRef] [PubMed]
19. Schmidt, D.; Thoden, U. Co-activation of the M. transversus auris with eye movements (Wilson's oculo-auricular phenomenon) and with activity in other cranial nerves. *Graefes Arch. Klin. Exp. Ophthalmol.* **1978**, *206*, 227–236. [CrossRef] [PubMed]
20. Leistritz, L.; Hochreiter, J.; Bachl, F.; Volk, G.F. Classification of facial movements in chronic facial palsy based on intramuscular EMG signals recorded from the paretic side. *Annu. Int. Conf. IEEE Eng. Med. Biol. Soc.* **2020**, *2020*, 662–665. [CrossRef] [PubMed]

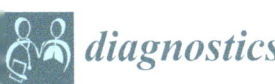

Case Report

Diagnostic Value of Preoperative Electrodiagnostic Analysis in a Patient with Facial Palsy and a Large Vestibular Schwannoma: Case Report

Myung Chul Yoo

Department of Physical Medicine and Rehabilitation, College of Medicine, Kyung Hee University Hospital, 23 Kyung Hee Dae-ro, Dongdaemun-gu, Seoul 02447, Korea; famousir@naver.com; Tel.: +82-2-958-8980; Fax: +82-2-958-8470

Abstract: Although radiologic methods confirm the diagnosis of patients with large vestibular schwannomas, these methods usually indicate only the size of the tumor and its possible nerve compression. Electrodiagnostic methods can reveal the functional state of the nerves, particularly the trigeminal and facial nerves, as well as providing a basis for objectively evaluating nerve injury. Due to the lack of an established objective evaluation method, electrodiagnostic methods were utilized to assess injury to the cranial nerve in a patient with a large vestibular schwannoma. A 79-year-old woman presented with a one-month history of right facial palsy, vertigo, dizziness, right postauricular pain, and right-sided hearing disturbance. Physical examination suggested injuries to the facial and vestibulocochlear nerves. Magnetic resonance imaging identified a vestibular schwannoma and showed that the tumor mass was affecting the brainstem, including the fourth ventricle, resulting in mild obstructive hydrocephalus. Preoperative electrodiagnostic evaluation identified asymptomatic trigeminal neuropathy accompanying a vestibular schwannoma. The patient underwent surgery, consisting of a suboccipital craniotomy with additional gamma knife radiosurgery. Postoperatively, she demonstrated significant recovery from right facial palsy and partial improvement of her neurologic symptoms. Large vestibular schwannomas with facial paralysis may be accompanied by additional entrapment neuropathy. Routine preoperative electrophysiological evaluation is recommended to establish a definitive diagnosis and evaluate the function of the trigeminal nerve, facial nerve, and brainstem in patients with large and compressive vestibular schwannomas.

Keywords: vestibular schwannoma; electrodiagnostic study; blink reflex; needle electromyography

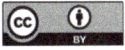

1. Introduction

Vestibular schwannomas, also called acoustic neuromas, are benign, slow-growing tumors that typically arise from the Schwann cells that form the vestibular portion of the vestibulocochlear nerve sheath [1]. These tumors are relatively common, accounting for 6–8% of all intracranial tumors and 80% of cerebellopontine angle (CPA) tumors [2,3]. Symptoms are usually associated with the compression of adjacent cranial nerves, the brainstem, and/or posterior fossa structures [4]. Although the most common symptoms of vestibular schwannoma are typically of insidious onset, other symptoms, including hearing deficits, tinnitus, vertigo, and dizziness, can occur. In addition, large tumors may compress the trigeminal nerve, resulting in trigeminal disturbances, such as hyperesthesia, paresthesia, and neuralgia. As a vestibular schwannoma grows, it can expand from its origin within the internal auditory canal (IAC) and extend into the brainstem or the CPA. The tumor can continue to enlarge and compress nearby cranial nerves. Clinically apparent facial paralysis is rare, occurring in fewer than 5% of patients with vestibular schwannoma, usually late in the course of disease [5,6]. In addition, a study of 1000 patients with vestibular schwannomas showed that 17% experienced trigeminal nerve disturbances, with major symptoms that included facial numbness (paresthesia), hypoesthesia, and pain [7].

Vestibular schwannomas must be large to affect the trigeminal or facial nerve. As the diagnosis is based on clinical findings, trigeminal nerve damage is not suspected unless patients report major symptoms, such as trigeminal neuralgia. At present, medical imaging, particularly magnetic resonance imaging (MRI), and physical examination are primarily used in the differential diagnosis of patients with neurological symptoms. Most vestibular schwannomas can be preoperatively diagnosed by MRIs that demonstrate tumor extension beyond the fundus into the proximal fallopian canal. Imaging has become crucial in initial screening and evaluation and can precisely characterize vestibular schwannomas, enabling surgical planning for their removal. However, the correlations of symptoms and tumor extensions with actual objective cranial nerve damage remain unclear, as are the ability to preoperatively determine the extent of damage to the cranial nerves and the clinical significance of this damage. As no other dependable diagnostic tools have emerged to evaluate nerve injuries, surgical exploration remains the only definitive method for establishing a diagnosis. Electrodiagnostic techniques, including evaluations of nerve conduction and blink reflex, and needle electromyography (EMG), may be objective and noninvasive methods for evaluating nerve injury in patients with vestibular schwannomas. This study describes the use of electrodiagnostic techniques to predict damage to the trigeminal and facial nerves in a patient with a large vestibular schwannoma.

2. Case Presentation

A 79-year-old woman visited the outpatient clinic of the Department of Otorhinolaryngology, Head and Neck Surgery of our university hospital with a 1-month history of right facial palsy, vertigo, dizziness, right postauricular pain, and right-sided hearing disturbance. Her medical history included bipolar hemiarthroplasty due to a right hip fracture, including total arthroplasty of both knees, in 2017. She had no history of neurological, psychological, or metabolic disorders. Physical and neurologic examinations revealed marked right peripheral facial palsy (House-Brackmann grade IV), gaze-evoked nystagmus, and cerebellar ataxic gait. No significant facial sensory deficit was observed. Based on her symptoms, injuries to her facial and vestibulocochlear nerves were suspected. Brain MRI showed a solid cystic mass with heterogeneous enhancement in the right CPA and IAC. The tumor measured 3.4 × 2.7 cm in size, with thin walls and high signal intensity similar to cerebrospinal fluid (CSF) on T2-weighted MRI images and low signal intensity on T1-weighted MRI images (Figure 1a,b). The extension of the tumor and brainstem distortion resulted in narrowing of the fourth ventricle and mild obstructive hydrocephalus due to the effect of the mass on the brainstem (Figure 1c).

The patient was referred to the Department of Physical Medicine and Rehabilitation for electrodiagnostic analysis to determine the extent of facial nerve injury and to plan surgical treatment. Electrodiagnostic methods included a nerve conduction study (NCS), assessment of blink reflex, and needle EMG, all of which were performed by a physical medicine and rehabilitation physician. The facial NCS recorded the latency and amplitude of the compound muscle action potential (CMAP) of the bilateral frontalis, orbicularis oculi, nasalis, and orbicularis oris muscles in response to stimulation of the temporal, zygomatic, and buccal branches of the facial nerve, respectively. The facial NCS showed delayed latency in all right-sided muscles, except for the orbicularis oculi, as well as a small CMAP amplitude in all right-sided muscles (Table 1).

The blink reflexes of the ipsilateral R1 and R2, and contralateral R2 potentials in response to stimulation of the supraorbital nerves bilaterally were recorded by surface electrodes placed over the orbicularis oculi muscles. Although left supraorbital nerve stimulation provoked normal ipsilateral R1 and R2 responses, it did not provoke a contralateral R2 response. In contrast, right supraorbital nerve stimulation did not induce ipsilateral R1 and R2 or contralateral R2 responses, indicating deficits in the afferent pathway of the right trigeminal nerve and the efferent pathway of the reflex arc, indicative of the facial nerve (Figure 2). A needle EMG examination of the bilateral frontalis, orbicularis oculi, nasalis, and orbicularis oris muscles innervated by the facial nerve was also performed. As right supraorbital nerve stimulation failed to produce potentials on either side, an additional needle EMG study of the bilateral masseter and temporalis muscles was performed to evaluate concomitant trigeminal neuropathy. All the right-sided muscles except for the nasalis muscle demonstrated fibrillation potentials, positive sharp waves, and abnormal motor unit action potential (MUAP) recruitment patterns, indicating subacute axonal loss (Table 1). All the left-sided muscles were normal on both the NCS and needle EMG examinations. Therefore, electrodiagnostic methods were able to confirm injury to both the trigeminal and facial nerves, allowing accurate documentation of the degree of axonal loss clinically in a patient with entrapment neuropathy resulting from compression by a large vestibular schwannoma.

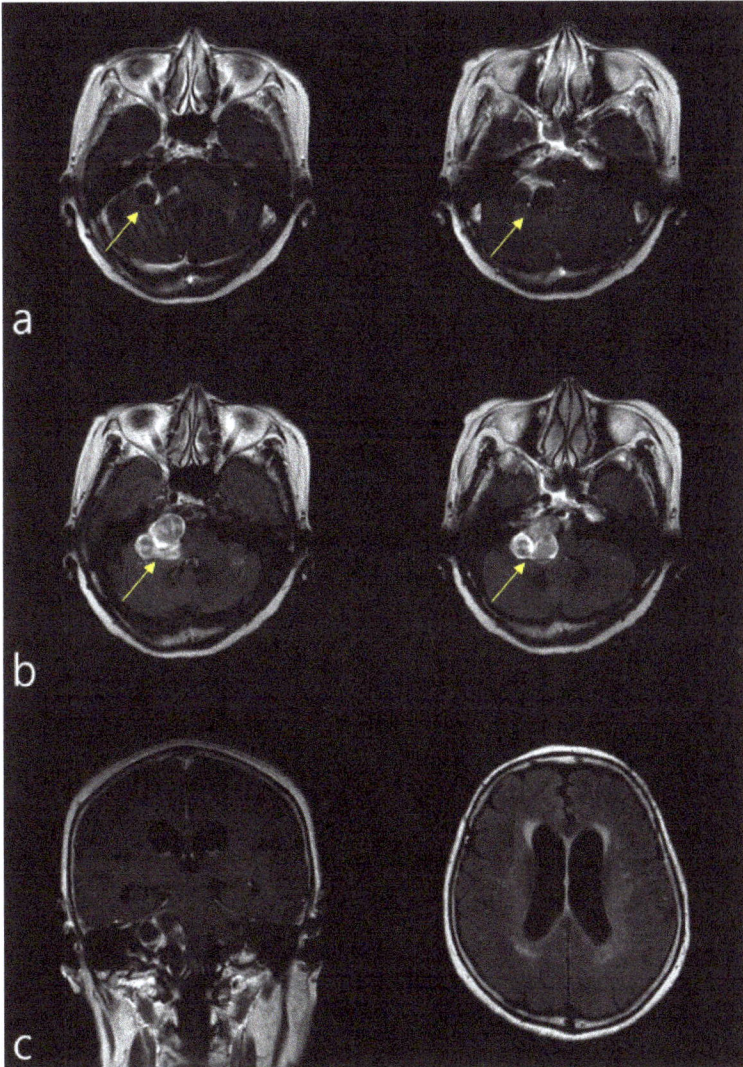

Figure 1. Brainstem magnetic resonance imaging (MRI). (**a**) T1-weighted enhanced imaging showing a well-margined, enhancing mass at the right cerebellopontine angle (3.4 × 2.7 cm), compatible with vestibular schwannoma (arrows). (**b**) T2-weighted MRI imaging, showing high signal intensity similar to CSF, demonstrating heterogeneous enhancement (arrows). (**c**) Image showing compression by the tumor mass of the right side of the brainstem, resulting in mild obstructive hydrocephalus.

Table 1. Results of the facial nerve conduction study and the needle EMG examination of the present patient.

Nerve and Sites	Latency (ms)	Amplitude (μm)	Duration (ms)	Area (mVms)
Rt. facial—Frontalis	3.90	246.7	3.90	1.0
Lt. facial—Frontalis	3.45	580.0	3.45	2.3
Rt. facial—Orbicularis oculi	2.85	305.0	2.85	1.2
Lt. facial—Orbicularis oculi	2.85	995.0	2.85	3.7
Rt. facial—Nasalis	3.55	188.3	3.55	0.6
Lt. facial—Nasalis	3.05	860.0	3.05	2.5
Rt. facial—Orbicularis oris	3.10	401.7	3.10	3.4
Lt. facial—Orbicularis oris	2.95	945.0	2.95	3.6

Muscle	Spontaneous Activity			MUAP		Recruitment Pattern
	IA	Fib	PSW	Amplitude	Duration	
Rt. Frontalis	normal	1+	2+	1−	normal	discrete
Lt. Frontalis	normal	none	none	normal	normal	normal
Rt. Orbicularis ocui	normal	1+	2+	normal	normal	discrete
Lt. Orbicularis ocui	normal	none	none	normal	normal	normal
Rt. Nasalis	normal	none	none	2−	normal	single unit
Lt. Nasalis	normal	none	none	normal	normal	normal
Rt. Orbicularis oris	normal	3+	3+	1−	normal	discrete
Lt. Orbicularis oris	normal	none	none	normal	normal	normal
Rt. Masseter	increased	2+	2+	2−	normal	discrete
Lt. Masseter	normal	none	none	normal	normal	normal
Rt. Temporalis	increased	2+	2+	1−	normal	reduced
Lt. Temporalis	normal	none	none	normal	normal	normal

Abbreviations: IA, insertion activity; Fib, fibrillation potentials; PSW, positive sharp waves; MUAP, motor unit action potential.

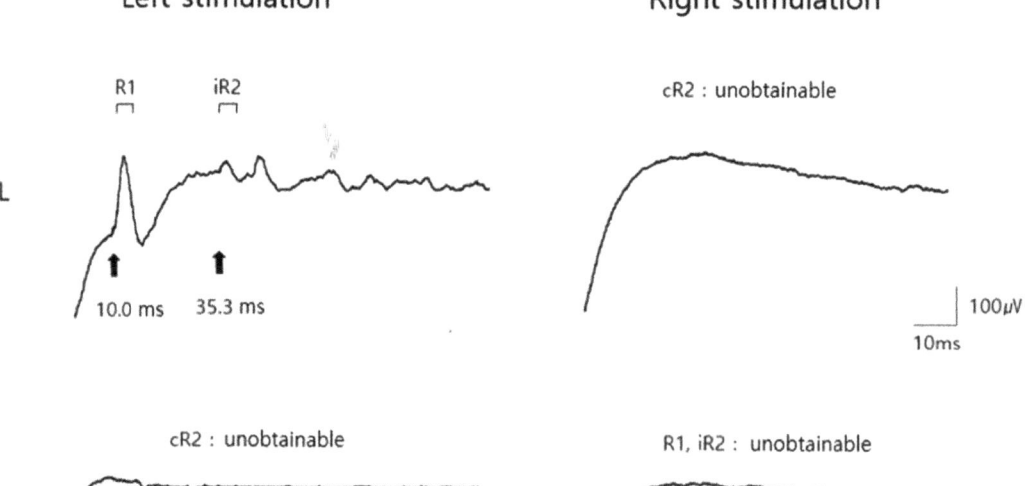

Figure 2. Preoperative blink reflex study results. Stimulation of the left supraorbital nerve provoked normal ipsilateral early wave (R1) and late wave (R2) responses, however did not provoke a contralateral R2 response. Stimulation of the right supraorbital nerve did not provoke ipsilateral R1 and R2 and contralateral R2 responses. Abbreviations: iR2, ipsilateral R2; cR2, contralateral R2.

One week later, the patient underwent retromastoid suboccipital craniotomy for tumor excision. Exposure of the lesion revealed that the tumor mass grossly compressed both the trigeminal and facial nerves. The patient experienced no postoperative complications, and postoperative histopathologic examination confirmed a vestibular schwannoma. The patient's neurologic symptoms were partially improved after surgery. However, a brain MRI performed one month after surgery revealed a remnant tumor mass near the right IAC. The patient underwent additional gamma knife radiosurgery for treatment of the remnant tumor. One month after gamma knife radiosurgery, the patient showed recovery from the right facial palsy (House–Brackmann grade II).

3. Discussion

Cystic vestibular schwannomas can appear on computed tomography or MRI as peripherally thin-walled tumors or centrally located thick-walled tumors. Although these tumors are benign, patients frequently experience rapid progression of facial nerve symptoms [8]. Clinical presentation is dependent on tumor size at diagnosis, the effect of the tumor mass on the brainstem, and possible obstruction of CSF pathways. In the present patient, severe brainstem displacement and fourth ventricle tumor compression resulted in mild hydrocephalus. Patients with large vestibular schwannomas, including those with stage IV tumors, therefore frequently present not only with auditory neuropathy and vestibulopathy, but also with entrapment nerve symptoms caused by pressure on the facial nerve. The incidence of symptoms and the anatomic relationship between the tumor and the respective cranial nerve have been described previously [9].

Generally, vestibular schwannoma-related trigeminal neuropathy is thought to be caused by direct pressure of the tumor on the trigeminal nerve, leading to demyelination of the somatosensory and pain fibers [5,10]. It has been estimated that 1–9.9% of patients with trigeminal neuralgia symptoms are eventually diagnosed with CPA tumors [11]. Although both cranial nerves in the present patient were directly compressed by the tumor, she lacked the classic provocative features associated with trigeminal neuropathy. Due to a lack of objective methods available to evaluate the cranial nerves, patients are usually diagnosed based on their subjective symptoms, such as facial paralysis, vertigo, dizziness, and hearing deficits. As the symptoms in the present patient were not as intense as expected for traditional trigeminal neuralgia, such as facial numbness, hypoesthesia, and pain, she was suspected of having facial and vestibulocochlear neuropathies.

Although MRI often confirms the diagnosis of cystic vestibular schwannomas, radiological findings may only indicate tumor size and the possibility of nerve compression, especially in patients with large tumors. In contrast, electrodiagnostic techniques including NCS, blink reflex, and needle EMG, can reveal the functional state of the nerves, particularly the trigeminal and facial nerves, and offer important information for the objective evaluation of nerve damage. Electrodiagnostic methods, such as NCS and EMG [12,13], have been used to assess the degree of facial nerve injury. These electrophysiologic techniques can indirectly quantify facial nerve function by recording the compound muscle action potentials (CMAPs) and motor unit action potentials (MUAPs) [14]. The degree of nerve degeneration can be estimated by comparing the peak-to-peak amplitudes of the CMAPs on the affected side with the response amplitudes on the non-affected side. Thus, extending electrophysiological assessment by evaluating the blink reflex or needle EMG of the facial muscles could indicate the actual degree of nerve and brainstem damage at the site of tumor compression [15].

Spontaneous waveforms recorded in resting muscles during needle EMG can be important in determining the type of underlying neuromuscular disorder and its severity, prognosis, and time course. Rapid insertion of the electrode into the muscle usually results in temporary electrical activity, which lasts slightly longer than the duration of electrode insertion, due to both direct physical stimulation and denervation of muscle fibers. Insertion activity usually does not last longer than 300 ms; activity that lasts more than 300 ms after the needle movement stops is abnormal and can be observed in cases of denervation, myopathy, and inflammation [16]. Damage to a nerve that innervates a muscle, as in denervation, can cause the muscle fiber to become hypersensitive and generate abnormal spontaneous discharge potentials, such as fibrillation or positive sharp waves. In general, abnormal spontaneous activity, including positive sharp waves and fibrillation potentials, suggests active denervation. This abnormality has been encountered in patients with various neuromuscular disorders that cause denervation or damage to muscle fibers [17]. In neuropathic diseases, recruitment is reduced and may be the earliest physiological sign of nerve injury. The MRI findings in the present patient showed the effect of the CPA tumor mass on the brainstem, including the fourth ventricle, resulting in mild obstructive hydrocephalus. In addition, damage to the loop of a reflex arc was evaluated by measuring the blink reflex, which can identify defects in afferent and efferent pathways. Moreover, the decreased CMAP amplitude of the facial NCS, abnormal spontaneous activity (insertion activity, fibrillation, and positive sharp waves), MUAP polyphasic pattern, and abnormal recruitment pattern of the needle EMG confirmed the subacute axonal loss of the two cranial nerves. Therefore, electrodiagnostic techniques confirmed injury to both the trigeminal and facial nerves in the present patient, indicating that electrodiagnostic methods allow accurate clinical documentation of the degree of axonal loss in patients with entrapment neuropathy resulting from compression by a large vestibular schwannoma.

Electrodiagnostic methods are generally more accurate than neurological tests in the diagnosis of facial neuropathies. For example, electrodiagnostic techniques were about five times more accurate at diagnosing facial neuropathy than clinical evaluations by neurologists [15]. Electrodiagnostic methods also allow accurate documentation of the state of the nerves and the degrees of axonal and demyelinating damage, making these methods both prognostic and diagnostic [18,19]. Interestingly, in the present patient, trigeminal neuropathy was preoperatively identified in a CPA tumor without neurological tests and symptoms of nerve compression. Electrodiagnostic methods, including evaluations of nerve conduction and blink reflex, and needle EMG, can objectively and noninvasively evaluate nerve injury in patients with vestibular schwannomas.

4. Conclusions

The findings in this patient indicate that additional entrapment neuropathy may be encountered in patients with large vestibular schwannomas and facial paralysis.

A routine preoperative electrophysiological evaluation can be helpful in the definitive diagnosis of nerve damage and can evaluate the function of the trigeminal nerve, facial nerve, and brainstem in patients with large and compressive vestibular schwannomas.

Funding: This research received no external funding.

Institutional Review Board Statement: The study was conducted in accordance with the guidelines of the Declaration of Helsinki and approved by the Institutional Review Board and Ethics Committee of Hyung Hee University Hospital (KHUH 2022-01-055, date of approval: 24 January 2022).

Informed Consent Statement: Informed consent was obtained from the patient involved in the study.

Data Availability Statement: Not applicable.

Acknowledgments: The authors thank the patient for allowing us to publish this case report.

Conflicts of Interest: The authors declare no conflict of interest.

References

1. Lin, E.P.; Crane, B.T. The Management and Imaging of Vestibular Schwannomas. *AJNR Am. J. Neuroradiol.* **2017**, *38*, 2034–2043. [CrossRef] [PubMed]
2. Tos, M.; Thomsen, J. Epidemiology of acoustic neuromas. *J. Laryngol. Otol.* **1984**, *98*, 685–692. [CrossRef] [PubMed]
3. Swartz, J.D. Lesions of the cerebellopontine angle and internal auditory canal: Diagnosis and differential diagnosis. *Semin. Ultrasound CT MRI* **2004**, *25*, 332–352. [CrossRef] [PubMed]
4. Espahbodi, M.; Carlson, M.L.; Fang, T.-Y.; Thompson, R.C.; Haynes, D.S. Small vestibular schwannomas presenting with facial nerve palsy. *Otol. Neurotol.* **2014**, *35*, 895–898. [CrossRef] [PubMed]

5. Matsuka, Y.; Fort, E.T.; Merrill, R.L. Trigeminal neuralgia due to an acoustic neuroma in the cerebellopontine angle. *J. Orofac. Pain* **2000**, *14*, 147–151. [PubMed]
6. Wexler, D.B.; Fetter, T.W.; Gantz, B.J. Vestibular schwannoma presenting with sudden facial paralysis. *JAMA Otolaryngol. Head Neck Surg.* **1990**, *116*, 483–485. [CrossRef] [PubMed]
7. Matthies, C.; Samii, M. Management of 1000 vestibular schwannomas (acoustic neuromas): Clinical presentation. *Neurosurgery* **1997**, *40*, 1–10. [PubMed]
8. Wu, H.; Zhang, L.; Han, D.; Mao, Y.; Yang, J.; Wang, Z.; Jia, W.; Zhong, P.; Jia, H. Summary and consensus in 7th International Conference on acoustic neuroma: An update for the management of sporadic acoustic neuromas. *World J. Otorhinolaryngol. Head Neck Surg.* **2016**, *2*, 234–239. [CrossRef]
9. Barker, F.G.; Jannetta, P.J.; Babu, R.P.; Pomonis, S.; Bissonette, D.J.; Jho, H.D. Long-term outcome after operation for trigeminal neuralgia in patients with posterior fossa tumors. *J. Neurosurg.* **1996**, *84*, 818–825. [CrossRef]
10. Jannetta, P.J. Arterial compression of the trigeminal nerve at the pons in patients with trigeminal neuralgia. *J. Neurosurg.* **1967**, *26*, 159–162. [CrossRef]
11. Shulev, Y.; Trashin, A.; Gordienko, K. Secondary trigeminal neuralgia in cerebellopontine angle tumors. *Skull Base* **2011**, *21*, 287–294. [CrossRef] [PubMed]
12. Esslen, E. The acute facial palsies: Investigations on the localization and pathogenesis of meato-labyrinthine facial palsies. *Schr. Neurol.* **1977**, *18*, 1–164.
13. Fisch, U. Maximal nerve excitability testing vs. electroneuronography. *Arch. Otolaryngol.* **1980**, *106*, 352–357. [CrossRef] [PubMed]
14. Mannarelli, G.; Griffin, G.R.; Kileny, P.; Edwards, B. Electrophysiological measures in facial paresis and paralysis. *Oper. Tech. Otolaryngol. Head Neck Surg.* **2012**, *23*, 236–247. [CrossRef]
15. Normand, M.M.; Daube, J.R. Cranial nerve conduction and needle electromyography in patients with acoustic neuromas: A model of compression neuropathy. *Muscle Nerve* **1994**, *17*, 1401–1406. [CrossRef] [PubMed]
16. Varma, S. Electromyography and neuromuscular disorders: Clinical-electrophysiologic correlations, edited by David, C. Preston and Barbara, E. Shapiro, 664 pp., Elsevier Saunders, 2012, $199. *Muscle Nerve* **2013**, *48*, 308. [CrossRef]
17. Rubin, D.I. Normal and Abnormal Spontaneous Activity. In *Handbook of Clinical Neurology*; Elsevier: Amsterdam, The Netherlands, 2019; Volume 160, pp. 257–279.
18. Jääskeläinen, S.K. The utility of clinical neurophysiological and quantitative sensory testing for trigeminal neuropathy. *J. Orofac. Pain* **2004**, *18*, 355–359. [PubMed]
19. Darrouzet, V.; Hilton, M.; Pinder, D.; Wang, J.-L.; Guerin, J.; Bebear, J.-P. Prognostic value of the blink reflex in acoustic neuroma surgery. *Otolaryngol. Head Neck Surg.* **2002**, *127*, 153–157. [CrossRef] [PubMed]

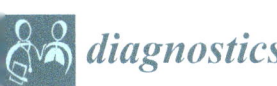

Article

Kabat Rehabilitation in Facial Nerve Palsy after Parotid Gland Tumor Surgery: A Case-Control Study

Ciro Emiliano Boschetti [1], Giorgio Lo Giudice [2,*], Chiara Spuntarelli [1], Carmine Apice [3], Raffaele Rauso [1], Mario Santagata [1], Gianpaolo Tartaro [1] and Giuseppe Colella [1]

[1] Oral and Maxillofacial Surgery Unit, Multidisciplinary Department of Medical-Surgical and Dental Specialties, University of Campania "Luigi Vanvitelli", Via Luigi de Crecchio, 6, 80138 Naples, Italy; ciroemilianoboschetti@gmail.com (C.E.B.); chiaraspunta@hotmail.it (C.S.); raffaele.rauso@unicampania.it (R.R.); mario.santagata@unicampania.it (M.S.); gianpaolo.tartaro@unicampania.it (G.T.); giuseppe.colella@unicampania.it (G.C.)
[2] Maxillofacial Surgery Unit, Department of Neurosciences, Reproductive and Odontostomatological Sciences, University of Naples "Federico II", Via Pansini, 5, 80131 Naples, Italy
[3] EY—AI & RPA Center of Excellence, Via Meravigli 12/14, 20123 Milan, Italy; carmine.apice@it.et.com
* Correspondence: giorgio.logiudice@unina.it

Abstract: Temporary facial nerve palsy after parotid tumor surgery ranges from 14 to 65%, depending on surgery, tumor type, and subsite. The study aimed to evaluate the role of Kabat physical rehabilitation in the outcomes of patients affected by severe facial nerve palsy following parotid gland surgery. The results and clinical data of two groups, Kabat and non-Kabat (control), were statistically compared. Descriptive statistics, the multiple linear regression model, difference in difference approach, and the generalized linear model were used. F-Test, Chi-square test, McFadden R-squared, and adjusted R-squared were used to assess the significance. The results showed that the House–Brackmann (HB) stage of patients who had physiotherapy performed were lower than the control group. The decrease of HB staging in the Kabat group at 3 months was −0.71 on average, thus the probability of having a high HB stage decreased by about 13% using Kabat therapy. The results are statistically significant, and indicated that when the Kabat rehabilitation protocol is performed, mainly in the cases of a high-grade HB score, the patients showed a better and faster improvement in postoperative facial nerve palsy.

Keywords: Kabat; facial nerve palsy; FNP; facial nerve paralysis; salivary gland surgery

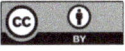

1. Introduction

Facial nerve palsy (FNP) is a disabling pathology that significantly affects the functional, psychological, social, and occupational aspects of a patient's life. This condition represents a frequent complication after parotid gland surgery, regardless of the surgical technique used and despite the most recent advances in surgical instrumentation and intraoperative monitoring [1,2]. The literature is unclear on the specific incidence of temporary FNP after parotid tumor surgery, and has been shown to range from 14 to 65% depending on the surgery, tumor type, and subsite [3,4].

In order to assess FNP severity, multiple scales have been developed such as the House–Brackmann (HB), Sunnybrook, or Yanagihara facial nerve grading scales [5,6]. The HB scale, which is the most adopted in the United States and Europe, is divided into six grades, from normal function to total palsy.

While the literature agrees that any treatment should be implemented as it overall improves the patients' quality of life, each to a different extent, no specific medical, surgical, or physiotherapy guidelines are currently available for post-operative FNP [7].

Updated guidelines have confirmed steroids to be effective at increasing the possibility of complete facial functional recovery in acute FNP, while novel treatments such as nimodipine and mycophenolate mofetile are under study. Nonetheless, postoperative corticosteroid treatment for iatrogenic FNP is unadvised, although clear evidence is lacking [8–11].

The literature describes the benefits of physiotherapy in nerve recovery (led either by a professional or home-based), and further studies have analyzed the aid given by facial taping and low-level laser therapy [12–15].

Kabat rehabilitation therapy is a treatment based on proprioceptive neuromuscular facilitation (PNF), a concept currently applied in orthopedic pathologies, post-stroke management, systemic sclerosis, and FNP rehabilitation [16–20]. This physiotherapy protocol is based on proprioceptors stimulation, by applying pressure in combination with traction movements, it is able to evoke and restore the neuromuscular circuits, recovering the normal function of the nerve endings in the muscles [21].

The aim of this study was to retrospectively evaluate the role of Kabat physical rehabilitation in the outcomes of patients affected by severe FNP following parotid gland surgery. Clinical data were compared between two different groups: a non-Kabat group and Kabat group.

2. Materials and Methods

This study was conducted retrospectively by evaluating the patients' medical reports treated at the Maxillo-Facial Surgery Unit of the University of Campania "Luigi Vanvitelli". The procedures were in accordance with the Helsinki Declaration, and the study was approved by the internal Ethical Committee (Prot. N. 313, 23 October 2020).

Patient records were selected according to the following inclusion criteria: patients with parotid gland tumor diagnosis, diagnosis of FNP after surgery, and HB stages IV-V recorded at 7 days follow-up.

The exclusion criteria were as follows: patients with preoperative facial palsy, patients that underwent postoperative radiotherapy, patients who started Kabat therapy more than seven days after surgery, patients with severe comorbidities, and/or those affected by pathologies that could interfere with the evaluation (neurodegenerative diseases or autoimmune diseases).

We collected clinical and pathological data (gender, age, pathology, tumor subsite, extent of surgery, and HB score) from 425 patients who underwent parotid gland surgery between January 2010 and March 2019 (Table 1).

Table 1. Patients demographics.

	No. (%)	Total Patients (n = 425)	HB IV (n = 34)	HB V (n = 22)
	Age (Years, Mean, Range)	46.7 (12–86)	47.4 (14–84)	63.9 (36–82)
Gender	Male	254	24	16
	Female	171	10	6
Pathology	Benign tumors	352	29	20
	Malignant tumors	73	5	2
Tumor subsite	Superficial to the facial nerve	293	21	7
	Deep to the facial nerve	47	6	6
	Superficial and deep location	85	7	9
Extent of surgery	Extracapsular dissection	184	7	1
	Partial parotidectomy	122	9	3
	Superficial parotidectomy	73	15	7
	Total parotidectomy	46	3	11

Out of 425 patients, 56 met our criteria: HB IV (34 subjects) and HB V (22 subjects). All subjects performed preoperative clinical examination, salivary glands ultrasonography, magnetic resonance imaging (MRI) with contrast enhancement, and fine-needle aspiration cytology with ultrasonography guide if indicated. The extent of surgery, extracapsular dissection (ED), partial parotidectomy (PP), superficial parotidectomy (SP), or total parotidectomy (TP) depended on the location, tumor size, and histological type. One head surgeon conducted the surgical procedures. Intraoperative facial nerve monitoring and surgical magnification using surgical loupes were used to identify the nerve. A single physician routinely evaluated the functional status of the facial nerve using the HB grading system at 7 days, and 1, 3, and 6 months post-operative. The evaluation was determined by measuring the excursion movements of the eyebrow and the angle of the mouth: 1 point was given for each 0.25 cm movement, to a maximum of 1 cm, and a final score ranging from 0 (total paralysis) to 8 points (normal function), which was then classified accordingly [5]. A physical rehabilitative protocol was employed according to the method proposed by Kabat, starting on day 7, at the time of suture removal, continuing three times per week for 12–24 weeks.

During the Kabat rehabilitation session, the patients performed specific diagonal and spiral movements, involving the following three muscle fulcrums:

- Upper fulcrum: includes the corrugators, frontalis, and orbicularis;
- Intermediate fulcrum: includes the common elevator muscle of the upper lip and wing of nose, the dilator naris, and the mitriform;
- Lower fulcrum: includes the risorius, zygomaticus major, the orbicularis, the zygomaticus minor, the triangular of the lower lip, buccinator, chin muscle, and square muscle of the chin [22].

The patients were split into two groups for the analysis: Kabat and non-Kabat (control). The former consisting of 28 of the 56 patients who had followed our therapeutic protocol and the latter consisting of patients who did not follow it, proceeding with standard therapies for the management of the rehabilitation cycle (28 patients). The two groups were homogeneous in terms of gender, age, HB grade, and extent of surgery, and we statistically compared the results and clinical data obtained (Table 2).

Table 2. Subject characteristics in the Kabat and non-Kabat (control) groups and House–Brackman score at 7 days (7 D), 1 month (1 M), 3 months (3 M), and 6 months (6 M). [a]: extracapsular dissection; [b]: partial parotidectomy; [c]: superficial parotidectomy; [d]: total parotidectomy).

Patient	Gender	Age	Extent of Surgery (E.D [a], S.P [b], P.P [c], P.T [d])	HB (7 D)	HB (1 M)	HB (3 M)	Hb (6 M)
				Kabat Group			
1	M	49	T.P	V	III	I	I
2	M	33	S.P	IV	III	II	I
3	M	52	P.P	V	IV	II	II
4	M	84	P.P	IV	IV	III	I
5	M	69	E.D	V	II	I	I
6	M	14	S.P	IV	IV	II	I
7	M	72	T.P	V	V	II	II
8	M	51	T.P	V	IV	III	III
9	M	37	S.P	IV	II	I	I
10	M	18	E.D	IV	I	I	I
11	M	76	S.P	V	IV	II	I
12	M	37	P.P	IV	I	I	I
13	M	41	T.P	IV	III	I	I
14	M	73	S.P	IV	IV	II	II
15	M	61	T.P	V	II	I	I
16	M	53	S.P	IV	II	I	I
17	M	76	E.D	IV	I	I	I
18	M	41	S.P	IV	III	II	II

Table 2. Cont.

Patient	Gender	Age	Exent of Surgery (E.D [a], S.P [b], P.P [c], P.T [d])	HB (7 D)	HB (1 M)	HB (3 M)	Hb (6 M)
19	M	55	S.P	IV	II	II	I
20	M	46	P.P	V	III	II	II
21	F	37	E.D	IV	II	I	I
22	F	68	T.P	IV	IV	II	I
23	F	71	S.P	V	II	I	I
24	F	48	P.P	IV	I	I	I
25	F	46	P.P	IV	II	I	I
26	F	47	S.P	IV	II	II	I
27	F	78	S.P	V	III	II	II
28	F	73	T.P	V	II	I	I
Non-Kabat Group							
1	M	45	P.P	IV	IV	III	I
2	M	36	S.P	V	V	III	II
3	M	65	P.P	IV	III	II	I
4	M	82	S.P	V	III	II	II
5	M	73	S.P	IV	IV	IV	I
6	M	16	E.D	IV	II	I	I
7	M	78	T.P	V	IV	II	II
8	M	54	T.P	V	III	III	III
9	M	39	S.P	IV	III	I	I
10	M	15	S.P	IV	II	I	I
11	M	78	T.P	V	IV	II	I
12	M	47	S.P	IV	II	II	I
13	M	29	S.P	IV	III	II	I
14	M	68	P.P	V	IV	III	I
15	M	57	T.P	V	III	II	II
16	M	66	S.P	IV	II	I	I
17	M	81	E.D	IV	III	II	I
18	M	33	P.P	IV	III	II	I
19	M	32	E.D	IV	IV	II	I
20	M	64	T.P	V	IV	III	III
21	F	19	E.D	IV	III	II	I
22	F	77	T.P	V	V	IV	II
23	F	65	S.P	V	IV	III	I
24	F	51	P.P	IV	III	II	I
25	F	32	S.P	IV	III	II	I
26	F	82	T.P	IV	IV	III	II
27	F	49	S.P	V	IV	IV	II
28	F	78	P.P	IV	II	I	I

Statistical Analysis

The statistical analysis and figures were produced using R (R Core Team, 2014). Descriptive statistic was used to evaluate the differences between the two groups and the relation between age and HB grading. A multiple linear regression model was adopted to evaluate a possible relationship between HB grade at 3 months and other variables present in our dataset. The difference in difference approach, typical of the Quasi-experimental design, was used to determine the effects of therapy on HB grading in both groups. F-Test and R-squared were used to assess the significance of our model. A logistic regression

model for binary data was used, dividing the variables of interest into the following two groups:
- People with a mild grading (from I to II) of HB registered at 3 months;
- People with a severe grading (from III to V) of HB registered at 3 months.

This model was further used considering two variables: age and Kabat therapy. Chi-square test and McFadden R-squared were used to assess the significance of our model.

3. Results

3.1. Descriptive Statistics

Kabat and non-Kabat (control) groups were homogeneous in terms of gender (20 males and 8 females), mean age (53.8 ± 18.3 vs. 54 ± 21.6), HB grade at 7 days, and extent of surgery. Our analysis was focused on the effects of Kabat considering the median position (3 months), as the other follow-up records could be perceived to be too close or too far from the surgical intervention. The graph shows that there are different compositions in HB grading, depending on whether the patients have followed Kabat therapy or not (Figure 1).

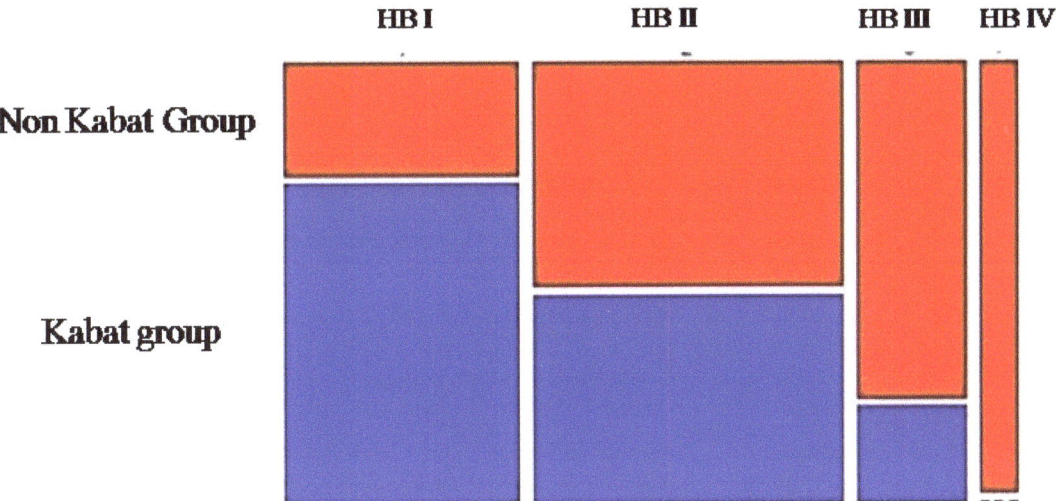

Figure 1. Graphical representation of the collected data.

The percentages of patients who had not used the therapy increased compared to the HB grading recorded. Regarding the relation between age and HB grading, it is possible to assume that postoperative recovery could be longer for older subjects than younger ones. A positive relation was shown: older people had a higher HB grading on average (Figure 2).

3.2. Multiple Linear Regression Model

The results of the multiple linear regression model showed the relation between the results and the Kabat therapy to be statistically significant ($p < 0.001$) (Table 3).

We grouped the extent of surgery variable, collapsing this in two levels, in order to divide people that received a total parotidectomy and those who did not. In this case, the extent of surgery was still not useful to explain our response variable. As the role played by the other variables was not significant, we decided to remove gender and extent of surgery from the dependent variables (Table 4).

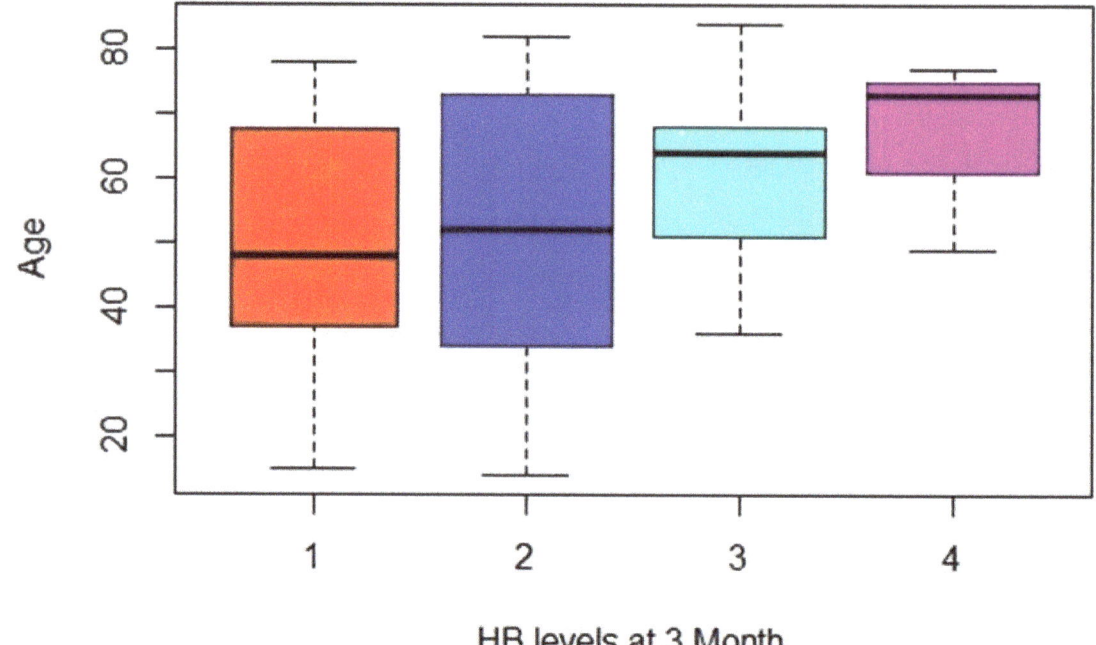

Figure 2. Graphical representation of the relation between age and HB score of the entire cohort of patients.

Table 3. Linear regression model with all variables [1] (EoS refers to different extent of surgery: PP, partial parotidectomy; SP, superficial parotidectomy; TP, total parotidectomy).

Parameter	Estimate	St.Error	t-Value	Pr (>|t|)	Level of Significance
Intercept	1.405911	0.423367	3.321	0.001701	**
Kabat	−0.712216	0.202041	−3.525	0.000929	***
Age	0.008280	0.005551	1.492	0.142208	
Gender	−0.049406	0.225573	−0.219	0.827539	
EoSPP [1]	0.449229	0.350219	1.283	0.205628	
EoSSP [1]	0.567987	0.314315	1.807	0.076894	
EoSTP [1]	0.593099	0.354328	1.674	0.100529	

** $p \leq 0.01$; *** $p \leq 0.001$; $p > 0.05$.

Table 4. Linear regression model with the final set of independent variables.

Parameter	Estimate	St.Error	t-Value	Pr (>|t|)	Level of Significance
Intercept	1.70734	0.31214	5.470	1.24×10^{-6}	***
Kabat	−0.71161	0.20144	−3.533	0.000862	***
Age	0.01070	0.00514	2.082	0.042151	*

* $p \leq 0.05$; *** $p \leq 0.001$.

The decrease in HB grading in the Kabat group at 3 months was −0.71 on average. The difference in difference approach result was almost identical to the one obtained with the linear regression model (−0.714286) ($p = 0.0006502$; adjusted R-squared = 0.2133).

Generalized Linear Model

The results of the logistic regression model are shown in Table 5.

Table 5. Logistic regression model for binary data results.

Parameter	Estimate	St.Error	Z Value	Pr (>|z|)	Level of Significance
Intercept	−2.37459	1.19865	−1.981	0.0476	*
Kabat	−2.03370	0.85060	−2.391	0.0168	*
Age	0.03181	0.01929	1.649	0.0992	

* $p \leq 0.05$; $p > 0.05$.

The odds ratio evaluation showed that the probability of having a high HB grading decreased by about 13% using Kabat therapy. Moreover, for each additional year of age, the odds of having a severe HB grading increased by about 3% ceteris paribus. The results were statistically significant, as shown by R-squared of McFadden (0.18) and Chi-Square tests ($p = 0.0057$).

Using the parameters obtained from the model and to provide a graphical intuition of the results, we plotted the profiles of the patients at different ages, using and not using Kabat therapy (Figure 3).

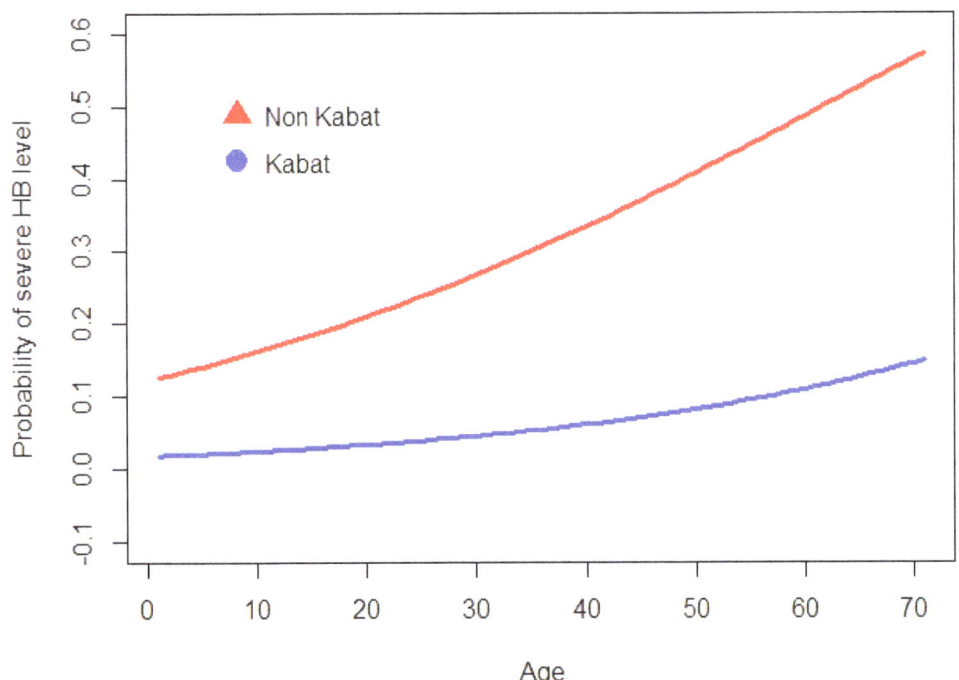

Figure 3. Profiles of patients at different ages using and not using Kabat therapy.

For example, at age 60, the probability of having severe facial nerve palsy (HB III, IV, or V at 3 months) is 0.08 if the patient follows Kabat therapy, while the same probability increases up to 0.39 if the patient does not (Figures 4 and 5).

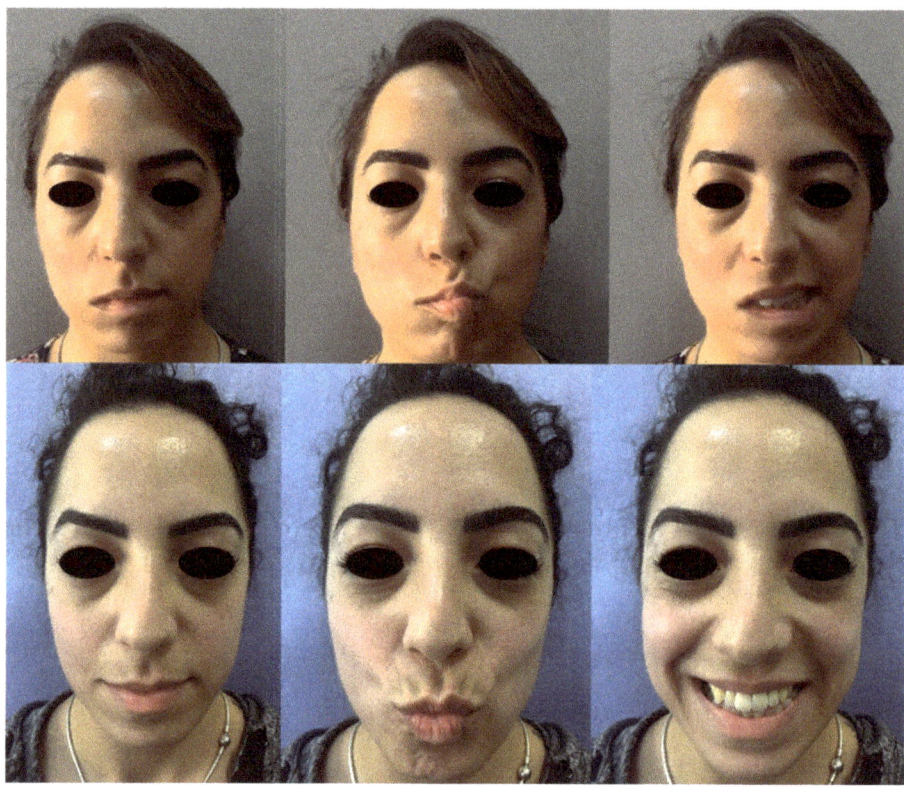

Figure 4. Patient 1. Clinical assessment of postoperative facial nerve palsy 7 days after surgery (**upper row**). Three month follow-up after Kabat therapy (**lower row**).

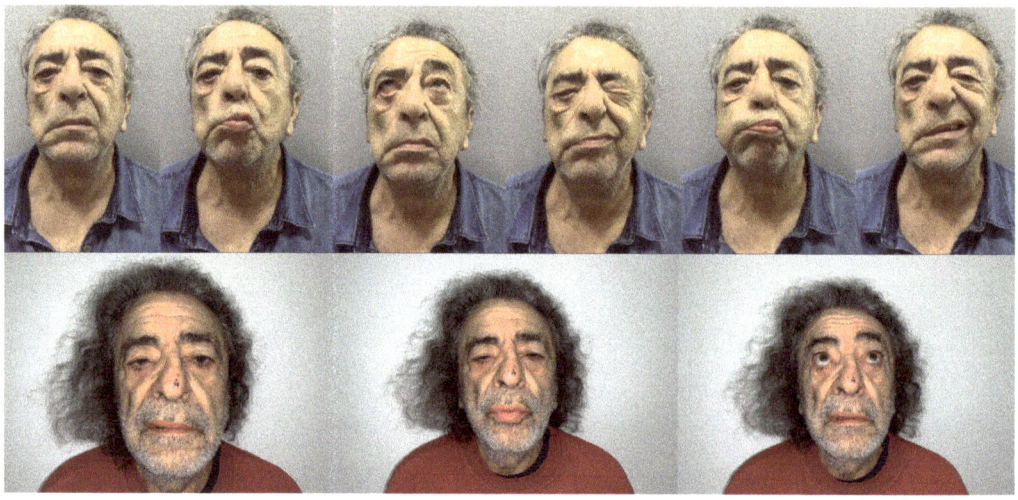

Figure 5. Patient 2. Postoperative facial nerve palsy 7 days after surgery (**upper row**) with noticeable right eye lagophthalmos. At the 3 month follow-up after Kabat therapy, right eye lagophthalmos was resolved (**lower row**).

4. Discussion

For head and neck surgeons, preservation of facial nerve integrity and function is a primary goal of parotid gland surgery, and still represents a major challenge. An occurrence of facial nerve palsy, despite the macroscopic continuity of the nerve, is not always tolerated, because of the possible impact on the quality of life, and the involvement of functional and aesthetic aspects (labial incontinence with drooling, chewing impairment, ectropion, keratoconjunctivitis, and severe facial asymmetry).

While authors have described the efficacy of Kabat rehabilitation in FNP from different etiologies, post-surgical studies are lacking. This study aimed to retrospectively evaluate the effects of the Kabat rehabilitation protocol that we routinely prescribed in patients with severe facial nerve deficiency (HB IV-V) after parotid gland surgery. A fair number of patients refused our physiotherapy prescription due to lacking financial resources to perform private therapy or no time available, thus allowing us to create a control group and evaluate the overall efficacy.

The facial nerve function was assessed and recorded 7 days, and 1, 3, and 6 months post-operative. The clinical outcomes recorded after 3 months could be considered the most interesting as they represent the median position compared to the other records (which could be considered either too close or too far from the surgery). Therefore, our analysis was focused mainly on the effects of Kabat at this time.

The graph in Figure 1 shows that there were different compositions in the grading of HB depending on whether the patients followed Kabat therapy or not. We observed that the percentages of patients who did not use the therapy increased compared to the HB grading recorded. This evidence supports the hypothesis that Kabat rehabilitation may have had, in statistical terms, a negative effect on the severity of facial nerve palsy.

The results shown in the multiple linear regression model and the difference in difference approach support the fact that rehabilitation is effective at decreasing high grading of HB (Tables 3 and 4). The results of the generalized linear model show that HB grading decreased when using Kabat therapy (Table 5).

In terms of our understanding of the effectiveness of the therapy, it is also valuable to mention that both the variables of age and Kabat had no significance and there was a less significant effect on the measurement of HB grading at six months. This drove us to the conclusion that, despite the fact that the recovery of the patients would occur in any case after a certain time, Kabat therapy can accelerate the recovery process.

After physical rehabilitation, the degree of improvement (grade reduction at the HB) was significant in comparison to the final condition of the control group. Most of the patients treated with rehabilitative therapy recovered fully (HB I), while for a significant part of the control group patients, the maximum recovery was HB II. Furthermore, considering the follow-up period, a substantial improvement in HB grading was already appreciated after 3 months in patients undergoing Kabat rehabilitation. In fact, 45% of HB V subjects had an outcome at HB I compared to the non-Kabat group, in which no one showed the same improvement.

When considering the role played by gender, the extent of surgery, and the improvement of HB grade, no relation was found in both groups (Table 3).

On the other hand, assessing the age of the patients, the rate and the time of recovery were influenced negatively. Several studies have shown similar results, finding that age is a reliable prognostic factor for the final outcome [23]. In both groups, the older patients showed a higher final HB grade and also a longer time of recovery, probably due to the obvious differences in face tone between young and old subjects [13]. The older rehabilitated patients recovered to a lower final grade, with a shorter time of recovery with respect to the non-Kabat patients of the same age.

The overall results show how the use of Kabat significantly reduced the severity of facial nerve palsy measured on the HB scale (Figure 3).

Kabat physical rehabilitation induced an increase in facial muscle tone in the affected side and on the contralateral one, with functional and esthetic improvements. The rehabilitation, as previously reported in the literature, when applied at an early stage, produced better and faster recovery [23].

In our study, excellent outcomes in rehabilitated patients already 3 months after surgery were observed, and early rehabilitative therapy was always recommended.

The patient must be psychologically supported and encouraged to follow post-operative therapeutic indications for rapid functional recovery [23–25]. Compliance to Kabat therapy is pivotal for its success, as it is for every physiotherapy regimen [26,27]. Moreover, as facial palsy may be impactful on the patients' social life, patients that notice substantial improvements between each follow-up are more prone to adhere to the physiotherapy regimen. Physicians may show comparison pictures and videos between follow-ups to let the patient acknowledge the improvements made, thus boosting the autonomous motivation and adherence to the therapeutic protocol. As a fair number of patients refused Kabat rehabilitation, we suggest providing an easily readable pamphlet, accompanied with explicative images, on how to perform Kabat therapy in a home-based fashion. We believe that such a compromise could be of help to patients and would promote satisfactory results, despite professional physiotherapy providing better outcomes.

Despite the promising results, this research had some limitations. The retrospective design of this study was chosen due to the availability of older HB scoring data in our database; lack of photo or video documentation for older cases did not allow us to perform a comparison using alternative, less subjective, scoring scales. The analysis provided by the House–Brackman scoring could be substituted using scoring systems such as Sunnybrook or eFace scale in further studies [6,28]. Facial nerve function analysis should provide both a static and dynamic evaluation of the condition. In fact, the Facial Nerve Grading Scale 2.0 was created as a revision of the HB scale, as a regional scale where the examiner assesses the function and synkinesis of four regions, which is then converted to a House–Brackmann scale grade, with consistent interobserver variability being reported [29]. Such low interobserver and intraobserver variability was also reported for the Sunnybrook Facial Grading Scale, retaining a high sensitivity and being able to track changes over time [30].

5. Conclusions

The results showed that early Kabat rehabilitation allowed for faster recovery of postoperative FNP diagnosed at any HB score. The improvement shown by patients affected by severe FNP (IV-V HB grade) suggests that early physiotherapy prescription might effectively reduce functional, aesthetic, and psychological sequelae.

Author Contributions: Conceptualization, C.E.B. and G.C.; methodology, R.R.; formal analysis, C.A.; investigation, C.S. and M.S.; writing—original draft preparation, C.E.B.; writing—review and editing, G.L.G.; supervision, G.T.; project administration, G.C. All authors have read and agreed to the published version of the manuscript.

Funding: This research received no external funding.

Institutional Review Board Statement: The study was conducted in accordance with the Declaration of Helsinki, and was approved by the Ethics Committee of University of Campania "Luigi Vanvitelli" (Prot. N. 313, 23 October 2020).

Informed Consent Statement: Informed consent was obtained from all subjects involved in the study. Written informed consent was obtained from the patients to publish this paper.

Data Availability Statement: Data are available upon reasonable request from the corresponding author (G.L.G).

Conflicts of Interest: The authors declare no conflict of interest.

References

1. Haring, C.T.; Ellsperman, S.E.; Edwards, B.M.; Kileny, P.; Kovatch, D.; Mannarelli, G.R.; Meloch, M.A.; Miller, C.; Pitts, C.; Prince, M.E.P.; et al. Assessment of Intraoperative Nerve Monitoring Parameters Associated With Facial Nerve Outcome in Parotidectomy for Benign Disease. *JAMA Otolaryngol. Head Neck Surg.* **2019**, *145*, 1137–1143. [CrossRef] [PubMed]
2. Eren, S.B.; Dogan, R.; Ozturan, O.; Veyseller, B.; Hafiz, A.M. How Deleterious Is Facial Nerve Dissection for the Facial Nerve in Parotid Surgery: An Electrophysiological Evaluation. *J. Craniofac. Surg.* **2017**, *28*, 56–60. [CrossRef] [PubMed]
3. Jin, H.; Kim, B.Y.; Kim, H.; Lee, E.; Park, W.; Choi, S.; Chung, M.K.; Son, Y.I.; Baek, C.H.; Jeong, H.S. Incidence of postoperative facial weakness in parotid tumor surgery: A tumor subsite analysis of 794 parotidectomies. *BMC Surg.* **2019**, *19*, 199. [CrossRef] [PubMed]
4. Bogart, K.R. Socioemotional functioning with facial paralysis: Is there a congenital or acquired advantage? *Health Psychol.* **2020**, *39*, 345–354. [CrossRef] [PubMed]
5. House, J.W.; Brackmann, D.E. Facial nerve grading system. *Otolaryngol. Head Neck Surg.* **1985**, *93*, 146–147. [CrossRef]
6. Berg, T.; Jonsson, L.; Engström, M. Agreement between the Sunnybrook, House-Brackmann, and Yanagihara Facial Nerve Grading Systems in Bell's Palsy. *Otol. Neurotol.* **2004**, *25*, 1020–1026. [CrossRef]
7. Luijmes, R.E.; Pouwels, S.; Beurskens, C.H.; Kleiss, I.J.; Siemann, I.; Ingels, K.J. Quality of life before and after different treatment modalities in peripheral facial palsy: A systematic review. *Laryngoscope* **2017**, *127*, 1044–1051. [CrossRef]
8. Min-Jung, O.T. Medical Management of Acute Facial Paralysis. *Otolaryngol. Clin. N. Am.* **2018**, *51*, 1051–1075. [CrossRef]
9. Gagyor, I.; Madhok, V.B.; Daly, F.; Sullivan, F. Antiviral treatment for Bell's palsy (idiopathic facial paralysis). *Cochrane Database Syst. Rev.* **2019**, *9*, CD001869. [CrossRef]
10. Kim, S.J.; Lee, H.Y. Acute Peripheral Facial Palsy: Recent Guidelines and a Systematic Review of the Literature. *J. Korean Med. Sci.* **2020**, *35*, e245. [CrossRef]
11. Varadharajan, K.; Beegun, I.; Daly, N. Use of steroids for facial nerve paralysis after parotidectomy: A systematic review. *World J. Clin. Cases* **2015**, *3*, 180–185. [CrossRef] [PubMed]
12. Infante-Cossio, P.; Prats-Golczer, V.E.; Lopez-Martos, R.; Montes-Latorre, E.; Exposito-Tirado, J.A.; Gonzalez-Cardero, E. Effectiveness of facial exercise therapy for facial nerve dysfunction after superficial parotidectomy: A randomized controlled trial. *Clin. Rehabil.* **2016**, *30*, 1097–1107. [CrossRef] [PubMed]
13. Monini, S.; Buffoni, A.; Romeo, M.; Di Traglia, M.; Filippi, C.; Atturo, F.; Barbara, M. Kabat rehabilitation for Bell's palsy in the elderly. *Acta Otolaryngol.* **2017**, *137*, 646–650. [CrossRef] [PubMed]
14. Di Stadio, A.; Gambacorta, V.; Ralli, M.; Pagliari, J.; Longari, F.; Greco, A.; Ricci, G. Facial taping as biofeedback to improve the outcomes of physical rehab in Bell's palsy: Preliminary results of a randomized case-control study. *Eur. Arch. Otorhinolaryngol.* **2021**, *278*, 1693–1698. [CrossRef]
15. Javaherian, M.; Attarbashi Moghaddam, B.; Bashardoust Tajali, S.; Dabbaghipour, N. Efficacy of low-level laser therapy on management of Bell's palsy: A systematic review. *Lasers Med. Sci.* **2020**, *35*, 1245–1252. [CrossRef]
16. Maddali-Bongi, S.; Landi, G.; Galluccio, F.; Del Rosso, A.; Miniati, I.; Conforti, M.L.; Casale, R.; Matucci-Cerinic, M. The rehabilitation of facial involvement in systemic sclerosis: Efficacy of the combination of connective tissue massage, Kabat's technique and kinesitherapy: A randomized controlled trial. *Rheumatol. Int.* **2011**, *31*, 895–901. [CrossRef]
17. Morreale, M.; Marchione, P.; Pili, A.; Lauta, A.; Castiglia, S.F.; Spallone, A.; Pierelli, F.; Giacomini, P. Early versus delayed rehabilitation treatment in hemiplegic patients with ischemic stroke: Proprioceptive or cognitive approach? *Eur. J. Phys. Rehabil. Med.* **2016**, *52*, 81–89.
18. Guiu-Tula, F.X.; Cabanas-Valdes, R.; Sitja-Rabert, M.; Urrutia, G.; Gomara-Toldra, N. The Efficacy of the proprioceptive neuromuscular facilitation (PNF) approach in stroke rehabilitation to improve basic activities of daily living and quality of life: A systematic review and meta-analysis protocol. *BMJ Open* **2017**, *7*, e016739. [CrossRef]
19. Tedla, J.S.; Sangadala, D.R. Proprioceptive neuromuscular facilitation techniques in adhesive capsulitis: A systematic review and meta-analysis. *J. Musculoskelet. Neuronal Interact.* **2019**, *19*, 482–491.
20. Gunning, E.; Uszynski, M.K. Effectiveness of the Proprioceptive Neuromuscular Facilitation Method on Gait Parameters in Patients With Stroke: A Systematic Review. *Arch. Phys. Med. Rehabil.* **2019**, *100*, 980–986. [CrossRef]
21. Kabat, H.; Knott, M. Proprioceptive facilitation therapy for paralysis. *Physiotherapy* **1954**, *40*, 171–176. [CrossRef] [PubMed]
22. Giacalone, A.; Sciarrillo, T.; Rocco, G.; Ruberti, E. Kabat rehabilitation for facial nerve paralysis: Perspective on neurokinetic recovery and review of clinical evaluation tools. *Int. J. Acad. Sci. Res.* **2018**, *6*, 38–46.
23. Robinson, M.W.; Baiungo, J. Facial Rehabilitation: Evaluation and Treatment Strategies for the Patient with Facial Palsy. *Otolaryngol. Clin. N. Am.* **2018**, *51*, 1151–1167. [CrossRef]
24. Ishii, L.E.; Godoy, A.; Encarnacion, C.O.; Byrne, P.J.; Boahene, K.D.; Ishii, M. What faces reveal: Impaired affect display in facial paralysis. *Laryngoscope* **2011**, *121*, 1138–1143. [CrossRef]
25. Bogart, K.; Tickle-Degnen, L.; Ambady, N. Communicating without the Face: Holistic Perception of Emotions of People with Facial Paralysis. *Basic Appl. Soc. Psych.* **2014**, *36*, 309–320. [CrossRef] [PubMed]
26. Jack, K.; McLean, S.M.; Moffett, J.K.; Gardiner, E. Barriers to treatment adherence in physiotherapy outpatient clinics: A systematic review. *Man Ther.* **2010**, *15*, 220–228. [CrossRef] [PubMed]
27. Lonsdale, C.; Hall, A.M.; Williams, G.C.; McDonough, S.M.; Ntoumanis, N.; Murray, A.; Hurley, D.A. Communication style and exercise compliance in physiotherapy (CONNECT). A cluster randomized controlled trial to test a theory-based intervention to

increase chronic low back pain patients' adherence to physiotherapists' recommendations: Study rationale, design, and methods. *BMC Musculoskelet. Disord.* **2012**, *13*, 104. [CrossRef]
28. Banks, C.A.; Jowett, N.; Azizzadeh, B.; Beurskens, C.; Bhama, P.; Borschel, G.; Coombs, C.; Coulson, S.; Croxon, G.; Diels, J.; et al. Worldwide Testing of the eFACE Facial Nerve Clinician-Graded Scale. *Plast. Reconstr. Surg.* **2017**, *139*, 491e–498e. [CrossRef]
29. Vrabec, J.T.; Backous, D.D.; Djalilian, H.R.; Gidley, P.W.; Leonetti, J.P.; Marzo, S.J.; Morrison, D.; Ng, M.; Ramsey, M.J.; Schaitkin, B.M.; et al. Facial Nerve Grading System 2.0. *Otolaryngol Head Neck Surg* **2009**, *140*, 445–450. [CrossRef]
30. Fattah, A.Y.; Gurusinghe, A.D.R.; Gavilan, J.; Hadlock, T.A.; Marcus, J.R.; Marres, H.; Nduka, C.C.; Slattery, W.H.; Snyder-Warwick, A.K.; Sir Charles Bell, S. Facial nerve grading instruments: Systematic review of the literature and suggestion for uniformity. *Plast. Reconstr. Surg.* **2015**, *135*, 569–579. [CrossRef]

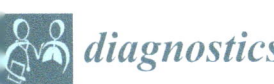

Case Report

Osteoradionecrosis of the Temporal Bone as a Rare Cause of Facial Nerve Palsy

Florian Schmidt [1,2,*], Katy Bradley [3,4] and Gerd Fabian Volk [5,6,7]

1. ENT Department, Portsmouth Hospitals University, Portsmouth PO6 3LY, UK
2. Klinik für HNO-Heilkunde, Evangelisches Krankenhaus Düsseldorf, 40217 Düsseldorf, Germany
3. Oncology Department, Portsmouth Hospitals University, Portsmouth PO6 3LY, UK; katy.bradley2@nhs.net
4. Oncology Department, Brighton and Sussex University Hospitals, Brighton BN2 5BE, UK
5. Department of Otorhinolaryngology, Jena University Hospital, Am Klinikum 1, 07747 Jena, Germany; fabian.volk@med.uni-jena.de
6. Facial-Nerve-Center Jena, Jena University Hospital, Am Klinikum 1, 07747 Jena, Germany
7. Center of Rare Diseases Jena, Jena University Hospital, Am Klinikum 1, 07747 Jena, Germany
* Correspondence: florian.schmidt@evk-duesseldorf.de

Abstract: We present a case of a 69-year-old male who presented with acute left facial nerve palsy, serous bloody otorrhea, otalgia, and exposed necrotic bone on the floor of his left ear canal. His medical history revealed a left canal wall-down (CWD) mastoidectomy thirty years ago. Subsequently, twenty years later, he received primary chemoradiotherapy for tonsil cancer on the same side. The patient's medical history, the typical clinical picture, and a comprehensive diagnostic workup, including imaging modalities and electrophysiology, finally led to a diagnosis of osteoradionecrosis of the temporal bone (ORNTB), with secondary facial nerve palsy. The facial nerve, unfortunately, did not recover and treatment remained conservative, as per the patient's preference. ORNTB is a rare, delayed complication after radiotherapy for head and neck cancer, which occurs after about 8 years and a minimum of 41.8 Gray of radiation to the affected area. Facial nerve palsy in ORNTB is rare, with only 2.9% of patients experiencing it, but, in our particular case, the patient had undergone an additional CWD mastoidectomy. The treatment options need to be personalized and aimed at symptom control. There should be awareness of the condition among ENT specialists, especially during head and neck cancer follow-ups, and in patients who have had mastoidectomy and radiotherapy affecting the ipsilateral temporal bone.

Keywords: facial nerve disorders; osteoradionecrosis; temporal bone; radiotherapy; head and neck cancer; mastoidectomy; surgery; facial palsy

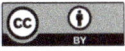

1. Introduction

Acute facial nerve palsy is, most commonly, an idiopathic condition (Bell's palsy). Other causes of facial nerve palsies include a wide range of disease processes, especially of the parotid gland and temporal bone. Thorough analysis of the patient's medical history, examination, and diagnostics are required to identify and treat the underlying condition. The following case reports on a rare condition, osteoradionecrosis of the temporal bone. This occurs several years post radiotherapy. It can affect the facial nerve, leading to facial nerve palsy. This case raises awareness of this rare condition among clinicians involved in facial nerve disorders, otology, and head and neck cancer treatment.

2. Case Description

A 69-year-old male was referred to our emergency ENT service with a three-week history of left facial nerve palsy. He also reported serous bloody otorrhea and ongoing otalgia. In primary care, he had already received 60 mg of prednisolone over ten days, amoxicillin and topical ciprofloxacin, alongside corneal protection.

Clinical examination revealed left lower motor neuron facial nerve paresis of a House-Brackmann grade V. The left ear showed widely exposed necrotic bone on the floor of the ear canal and over the facial ridge towards the mastoid cavity, with debris (Figure 1).

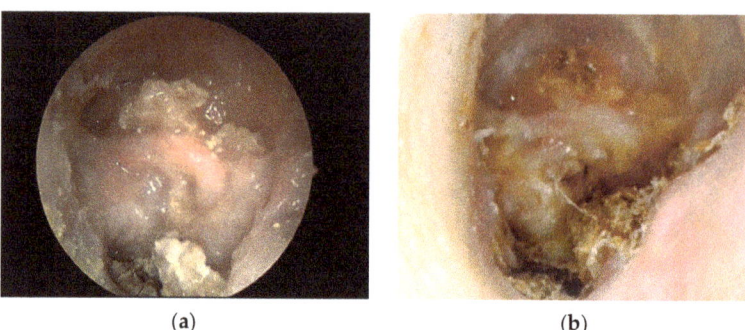

(a)   (b)

Figure 1. Left ear canal and mastoid cavity at initial presentation (**a**) and after six months, (**b**) with persistent, widely exposed necrotic bone on the floor of the external auditory meatus, facial ridge, and debris.

His medical history revealed a left canal wall-down (CWD) mastoidectomy about thirty years ago. Subsequently, twenty years later (ten years ago), a left-sided squamous cell carcinoma of his tonsil was diagnosed, staged T3N1M0 (7th Edition of the AJCC TNM staging system). He underwent curativeinduction chemotherapy, including fluorouracil, docetaxel, and cisplatin, followed by a radiation dose of 66 Gray (Gy) to his left oropharynx and neck, with concurrent cisplatin (Figure 2). Seven years after his tonsil cancer, he had complained of intermittent otalgia and discomfort in his left periauricular, and was treated with microsuction and topical antibiotics for suspected mastoid cavity infections. Further review of his medical history revealed type II diabetes mellitus, which was medicated orally with diabetic retinopathy and peripheral neuropathy.

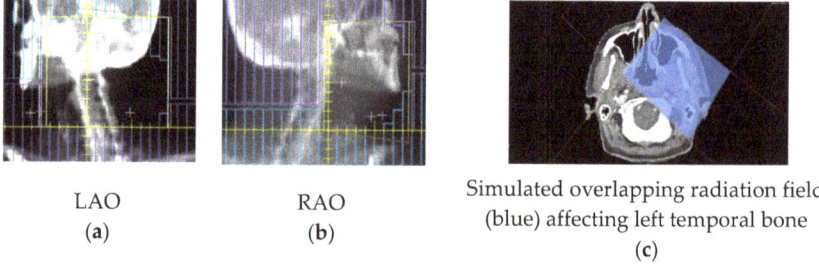

LAO   RAO   Simulated overlapping radiation field
(**a**)   (**b**)   (blue) affecting left temporal bone
                                               (**c**)

Figure 2. Upper radiation fields with 66 Gray (Gy) in 33 fractions to the left oropharynx tumor and neck. Radiotherapy was planned with 3D conformal radiotherapy, utilizing two fields to the upper volume: left anterior oblique (LAO) (**a**) and right anterior oblique (RAO) (**b**) fields, and the beam's eye radiographs shown. These fields have been reconstructed on axial CT, to indicate the approximate volume (**c**). The area where the fields overlap (blue) received 66 Gy.

At this point, the considered differential diagnosis included complicated acute otitis media, recurrent cholesteatoma, and malignancy of the middle ear and/or external auditory canal. Initially, however, the main diagnosis was thought to be malignant otitis externa (MOE), considering his diabetes.

The following work-up included microbiology from the ear, which revealed no bacterial growth, but some Candida species. A tissue biopsy from the ear canal reported hyperkeratosis, without significant inflammation, fungal organisms, dysplasia, or malignancy. His pure-tone audiogram revealed severe-to-profound pantonal hearing loss on the left (85–110 dB) and presbycusis (10–70 dB) on the right. He then underwent computed tomography (CT) scanning of his petrous bones and neck, reporting non-specific soft tissue in the mastoid cavity, post-surgical changes after previous CWD mastoidectomy, with removal of the ossicular chain, and patchy bony erosion of the external ear canal floor, as well as fatty changes in the left parotid gland, as compared to the right. There were normal appearances of the inner ear structures and the right temporal bone, and there was no evidence of local tumor recurrence or metastatic disease. A technetium uptake scan reported increased osteoblastic activity around the bony portion of the left external auditory canal. Magnetic resonance imaging (MRI) showed enhancement of the left facial nerve and small traces of diffusion in isointense/hyperintense material that was present, which involved the operated left mastoid cavity along the roof, floor, and medial aspect (Figure 3).

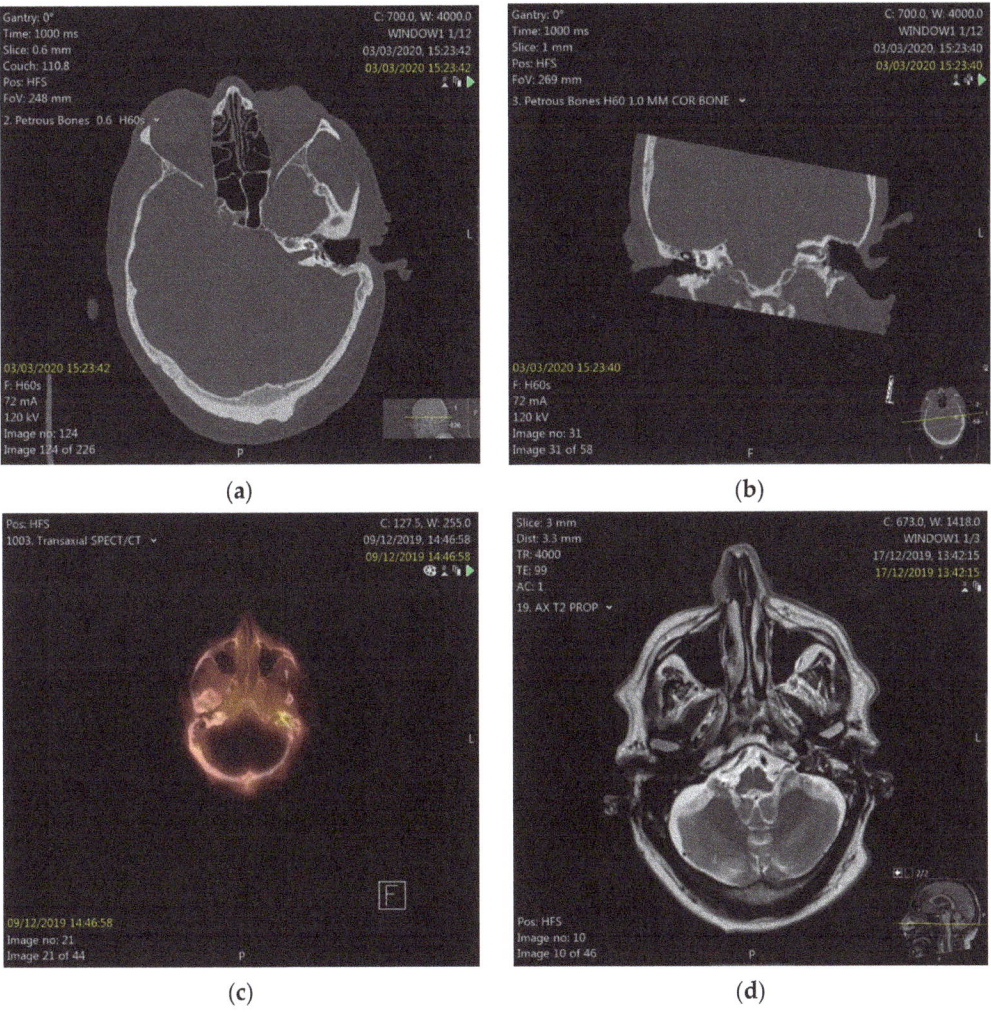

Figure 3. Computed tomography (CT) of petrous bones in axial (**a**) and coronal (**b**) planes, showing a situation after the left canal wall-down mastoidectomy, with patchy bony erosion of the floor of the external auditory meatus (white arrow) and uncovered facial nerve. Nuclear medicine scan (**c**) showing uptake around the left EAM. Magnetic resonance imaging (MRI) showing enhancement of the left mastoid (**d**).

He was commenced on a local MOE protocol with oral ciprofloxacin and intravenous ceftazidime for a total of six weeks, and received careful aural toilet and corneal protection. His diabetes was treated with insulin.

After completing treatment, his facial nerve did improve to House–Brackmann grade IV, and the ear was dry and pain free. A needle electromyography only revealed very limited voluntary facial muscle activity in the left orbicularis oculi muscle and no voluntary motor unit activity in any other tested facial muscle on the left side of the face, but also showed no signs of denervation.

Altogether, symptom control was achieved, leaving residual facial nerve palsy and persistent exposed necrotic bone in the ear canal. Based on his medical history, and subsequent investigations, the diagnosis of osteoradionecrosis of the temporal bone (ORNTB), with secondary facial nerve palsy, was established. It must be noted that the correct diagnosis was reached only three years after the development of the first symptoms. At that point, surgery, in the form of subtotal petrosectomy with vascularised flap obliteration, was offered, but, due to comorbidities and the patient's preference, conservative management was pursued, with regular aural care.

3. Discussion

Osteoradionecrosis of the temporal bone after radiotherapy (RT) was first described in 1926 as bony osteitis [1]. It is believed to be "due to radiation damage to blood vessels, causing osteocyte loss, fibrosis, hypocellularity and fatty degeneration of bone" [2]. The tympanic bone seems to be susceptible to radiation effects because of its "superficial position, thin epithelium and resident flora" [3]. A systematic review, including thirty-eight studies, encompassing 364 patients with ORNTB, reported that the mean lag time between radiotherapy and ORN symptoms was 7.9 years (range 6 months to 48 years) [3,4]. The most commonly radiated primary sites leading to the condition were the nasopharynx (36.8%), parotid (20.2%), and external auditory canal (16.3%) [4], unlike our case of an oropharynx primary. The mean radiation dose to the affected temporal bone was reported as 53.1 Gy, with a minimum of 41.8 Gy [3].

Despite differences in the initial treatment approaches for advanced stage III/IV head and neck cancers (especially oropharynx primaries, as described here), such as primary surgery, being more common in Europe and Germany compared to the United States and the United Kingdom, where organ preservation primary chemoradiation protocols are more often employed [5,6], radiation therapy plays a crucial part in the multimodal management of these tumors. The doses of curative primary radiation to gross tumor sites have to exceed 60 Gy (usually a dose equivalent of 70 Gy in 35 fractions), and even elective volumes in the neck range between 30 and 60 Gy. Postoperative radiation to high-risk areas employs volumes between 60 and 66 Gy. Furthermore, in the Anglo-American region, even early-stage oropharyngeal tumors (T1, T2) might be treated with radical radiation as a single modality.

The key clinical finding in ORNTB is visible, exposed necrotic bone in the external auditory canal [3]. Other common symptoms are otorrhea (33.3%), hearing loss (29.1%) and otalgia (17%) [4]. In contrast, facial nerve palsy, as a feature of ORNTB, is rarely reported, with only 2.9% reported cases in a large review [4]. This is likely due to the deep, bony protected course of the facial nerve within the temporal bone. In our case, we think that altered anatomy after the previous CWD mastoidectomy was a risk factor, with bony erosion leading to an exposed facial nerve in the mastoidal segment and subsequent nerve damage.

Facial nerve palsy was the critical symptom in our case, initiating the described comprehensive diagnostic procedure, which was needed to finally reach the correct diagnosis. For acute lower facial nerve palsies, there is no international standard for the optimal extend of diagnostics. However, for ENT specialists, a thorough clinical examination of the ear and parotid gland should be mandatory. Furthermore, the degree of facial nerve impairment should be recorded, which, in clinical routine, is often conducted using subjective measures, such as the House–Brackmann Scale or the Sunnybrook Facial Grading Scale, as objective means, like automated image analysis tools, are still being developed. Electromyography in this context can be helpful in delineating the degree of facial nerve injury and in monitoring the condition. CT scanning of the temporal bone as initial imaging provided, in our case, important information about the regional bony anatomy and extent of disease. Nuclear medicine uptake scans, often used to monitor the treatment response for malignant otitis externa, can provide information about acute inflammation via the accumulation of tracers in the inflamed area. Finally, MRI scanning was rather unspecific for ORNTB, but was helpful in this case to exclude other causes of non-recovering facial nerve palsy.

Different classification systems of ORNTB have been introduced. In 1975, Ramsden et al. distinguished between localized disease, confined to the EAC and tympanic bone, with mild otalgia and otorrhea, and diffuse disease, with extensive necrosis of the temporal bone, with involvement of adjacent structures, such as the labyrinth, facial nerve, TMJ, or brain, with severe otalgia and profuse otorrhea [7]. In 2011, Morrissey and Grigg established a classification system of ORNTB, ranging from grade I (erosion of the EAC skin, without bony involvement) to IVb (skull base involvement) [8]. Finally, in 2014, Kammeijer, in his classification, divided localized disease and diffuse type A, with extensive necrosis of the temporal bone, with involvement of adjacent structures, but little pain and intact hearing, as well as diffuse type B, with similar features, but severe pain and infection and/or no functional hearing [9]. Our presented case certainly fell into a more severe category of diffuse disease with cranial nerve involvement.

There is currently a lack of randomized controlled trials regarding the condition, and, therefore, treatment needs to be personalized and aimed towards symptom control. The management options are wide ranging, including topical/systemic anti-microbiologic treatment, hyperbaric oxygen therapy, analgesia, debridement, and, in more severe cases, surgery in the form of lateral temporal bone resection, mastoidectomy, or subtotal petrosectomy, plus or minus flap obliteration [3,4]. In one study regarding parotid malignancies, interestingly, ORNTB after parotidectomy and RT was found in 1.9% of cases, but after parotidectomy, mastoidectomy and RT, it was found in 12.5%, and after combined parotidectomy, subtotal petrosectomy, and flap obliteration of the mastoid cavity and RT, it was found in 0% [10]. Generally, there seems to be consensus that in localized ORNTB with minor symptoms, nonsurgical (conservative) therapy is appropriate, but in patients with diffuse disease, cases refractory to conservative measures or major symptoms, surgery is more likely to be required [11]. The role of hyperbaric oxygen therapy in ORNTB is controversial. It may be considered as an adjunct, but a lack of evidence of its efficacy remains [11]. The outcomes of localized disease, which were treated conservatively, reported adequate resolution of symptoms in 89% of cases [4]. In the surgical group, the systematic literature review by Yuhan et al. described 93.8% of the subtotal of petrosectomies, 90.9% of lateral temporal bone resections, and 59.76% of mastoidectomies as successfully achieving the treatment goals [4]. Kammeijer et al. also proposed, in particular, subtotal petrosectomy, with a success rate of 90.9%, with vascularized flap obliteration [9].

The options for long-standing facial nerve rehabilitation are complex, including physical therapy and various surgical reanimation procedures [12]. These need to be scheduled in the context of the management of the underlying ORNTB and patients' factors.

With evidence for treatments of the disease remaining currently limited, primary prevention should be taken into consideration. This would include particularly vascularised soft tissue reconstruction after ablative oncological procedures, avoiding tension over the temporal bone, and ensuring that no exposed bone is present within the radiation field at the beginning of radiotherapy. Finally, it has to be highlighted that in this case, RT was still planned with 3D conformal radiotherapy. New developments of intensity-modulated radiotherapy (IMRT), which is now established as a modern technique of radiation therapy, allow better control of radiation dose delivery in the head and neck. This has been shown to reduce, especially, radiation-induced xerostomia by sparing of salivary glands [13]. One hopes that ORNTB might be reduced as well in the future, through sparing of critical (exposed) bony structures.

Furthermore, the patient had a history of diabetes, with retinopathy and neuropathy. It is known that poor glycaemic control is associated with increased wound infections and postoperative morbidity, and, therefore, in head and neck cancer patients, optimization of diabetes is advised peri-operatively [14]. However, diabetic neuropathy, in contrast to an isolated facial nerve (motor) dysfunction, typically causes sensory dysfunction and pain, beginning distally in the lower extremities [15]. It has been reported that the incidence of cranial nerve palsies (including CN VII) is higher in diabetic patients, compared to non-diabetics; however, isolated cranial nerve VII palsies seem to be less closely related to diabetic complications than, for example, oculomotor neuropathies [16]. Therefore, diabetes, in the setting of clinically present ORNTB, might have been a contributary factor, but was, altogether, difficult to ascertain. Additionally, chemotherapy did employ fluorouracil, docetaxel and cisplatin in this case. Both docetaxel and cisplatin, and especially their combination, have been shown to frequently predominantly cause peripherally (lower and upper limbs) sensory neuropathies, but also motor neuropathies, usually within weeks of treatment [17,18]. Even though chemotherapy-induced neuropathies can progress after the completion of treatment, as the onset of the facial nerve dysfunction occurred more than seven years after chemotherapy, the influence of both drugs as causative agents appears unlikely in this case.

4. Conclusions

Osteoradionecrosis of the temporal bone is a delayed complication. It occurs several years after RT for head and neck cancer, and is a rare cause of facial nerve palsy. It is important to consider the diagnosis in patients with a history of mastoidectomy and RT affecting the ipsilateral temporal bone.

Funding: This research received no external funding.

Institutional Review Board Statement: I confirm adherence to ethical guidelines. Case series of up to 3 or fewer patients with de-identified data are exempt from IRB approval requirements as per the University of Arkansas IRB board.

Informed Consent Statement: Informed consent was obtained from all subjects involved in the study. Written informed consent has been obtained from the patient(s) to publish this paper.

Data Availability Statement: Not applicable.

Conflicts of Interest: The authors declare no conflict of interest.

References

1. Ewing, J. Radiation Osteitis. *Acta Radiol.* **1926**, *6*, 399–412. [CrossRef]
2. Marx, R.E. Osteoradionecrosis: A new concept of its pathophysiology. *J. Oral Maxillofac. Surg.* **1983**, *41*, 283–288. [CrossRef]
3. Sharon, J.D.; Khwaja, S.S.; Drescher, A.; Gay, H.; Chole, R.A. Osteoradionecrosis of the temporal bone: A case series. *Otol. Neurotol.* **2014**, *35*, 1207–1217. [CrossRef] [PubMed]
4. Yuhan, B.T.; Nguyen, B.K.; Svider, P.F.; Raza, S.N.; Hotaling, J.; Chan, E.; Hong, R.S. Osteoradionecrosis of the Temporal Bone: An Evidence-Based Approach. *Otol. Neurotol.* **2018**, *39*, 1172–1183. [CrossRef] [PubMed]
5. Hermanns, I.; Ziadat, R.; Schlattmann, P.; Guntinas-Lichius, O. Trends in Treatment of Head and Neck Cancer in Germany: A Diagnosis-Related-Groups-Based Nationwide Analysis, 2005–2018. *Cancers* **2021**, *13*, 6060. [CrossRef] [PubMed]
6. Johnson, D.E.; Burtness, B.; Leemans, C.R.; Lui VW, Y.; Bauman, J.E.; Grandis, J.R. Head and neck squamous cell carcinoma. *Nat. Rev. Dis. Primers* **2020**, *6*, 92. [CrossRef] [PubMed]
7. Ramsden, R.T.; Bulman, C.H.; Lorigan, B.P. Osteoradionecrosis of the temporal bone. *J. Laryngol. Otol.* **1975**, *89*, 941–955. [CrossRef] [PubMed]
8. Morrissey, D.; Grigg, R. Incidence of osteoradionecrosis of the temporal bone. *ANZ J. Surg.* **2011**, *81*, 876–879. [CrossRef] [PubMed]
9. Kammeijer, Q.; van Spronsen, E.; Mirck, P.G.; Dreschler, W.A. Treatment outcomes of temporal bone osteoradionecrosis. *Otolaryngol. Head Neck Surg.* **2015**, *152*, 718–723. [CrossRef] [PubMed]

10. Leonetti, J.P.; Marzo, S.J.; Zender, C.A.; Porter, R.G.; Melian, E. Temporal bone osteoradionecrosis after surgery and radiotherapy for malignant parotid tumors. *Otol. Neurotol.* **2010**, *31*, 656–659. [CrossRef] [PubMed]
11. Herr, M.W.; Vincent, A.G.; Skotnicki, M.A.; Ducic, Y.; Manolidis, S. Radiation Necrosis of the Lateral Skull Base and Temporal Bone. In *Seminars in Plastic Surgery*; Thieme Medical Publishers, Inc.: New York, NY, USA, 2020; Volume 34, pp. 265–271. [CrossRef]
12. Jowett, N.; Hadlock, T.A. A Contemporary Approach to Facial Reanimation. *JAMA Facial Plast. Surg.* **2015**, *17*, 293–300. [CrossRef] [PubMed]
13. Nutting, C. Radiotherapy in head and neck cancer management: United Kingdom National Multidisciplinary Guidelines. *J. Laryngol. Otol.* **2016**, *130*, S66–S67. [CrossRef] [PubMed]
14. Robson, A.; Sturman, J.; Williamson, P.; Conboy, P.; Penney, S.; Wood, H. Pre-treatment clinical assessment in head and neck cancer: United Kingdom National Multidisciplinary Guidelines. *J. Laryngol. Otol.* **2016**, *130*, S13–S22. [CrossRef] [PubMed]
15. Feldman, E.L.; Callaghan, B.C.; Pop-Busui, R.; Zochodne, D.W.; Wright, D.E.; Bennett, D.L.; Bril, V.; Russell, J.W.; Viswanathan, V. Diabetic neuropathy. *Nat. Rev. Dis. Primers* **2019**, *5*, 41. [CrossRef] [PubMed]
16. Watanabe, K.; Hagura, R.; Akanuma, Y.; Takasu, T.; Kajinuma, H.; Kuzuya, N.; Irie, M. Characteristics of cranial nerve palsies in diabetic patients. *Diabetes Res. Clin. Pract.* **1990**, *10*, 19–27. [CrossRef]
17. Hilkens, P.H.; Pronk, L.C.; Verweij, J.; Vecht, C.J.; van Putten, W.L.; van den Bent, M.J. Peripheral neuropathy induced by combination chemotherapy of docetaxel and cisplatin. *Br. J. Cancer* **1997**, *75*, 417–422. [CrossRef] [PubMed]
18. Starobova, H.; Vetter, I. Pathophysiology of Chemotherapy-Induced Peripheral Neuropathy. *Front. Mol. Neurosci.* **2017**, *10*, 174. [CrossRef] [PubMed]

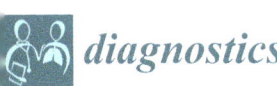

Article

Facial Emotion Recognition in Patients with Post-Paralytic Facial Synkinesis—A Present Competence

Anna-Maria Kuttenreich [1,2,3,4,5,*], Gerd Fabian Volk [1,2,3], Orlando Guntinas-Lichius [1,2,3], Harry von Piekartz [6] and Stefan Heim [4,5,7]

1. Department of Otorhinolaryngology, Jena University Hospital, Am Klinikum 1, 07747 Jena, Germany; fabian.volk@med.uni-jena.de (G.F.V.); orlando.guntinas@med.uni-jena.de (O.G.-L.)
2. Facial-Nerve-Center Jena, Jena University Hospital, Am Klinikum 1, 07747 Jena, Germany
3. Center of Rare Diseases Jena, Jena University Hospital, Am Klinikum 1, 07747 Jena, Germany
4. Department of Psychiatry, Psychotherapy and Psychosomatics, Medical Faculty, RWTH Aachen University, Pauwelsstr. 30, 52074 Aachen, Germany; sheim@ukaachen.de
5. Department of Neurology, Medical Faculty, RWTH Aachen University, Pauwelsstr. 30, 52074 Aachen, Germany
6. Department of Physical Therapy and Rehabilitation Science, Osnabrück University of Applied Sciences, Albrechtstr. 30, 49076 Osnabrück, Germany; h.von-piekartz@hs-osnabrueck.de
7. Institute of Neuroscience and Medicine (INM-1), Forschungszentrum Jülich, Leo-Brand-Strasse 5, 52428 Jülich, Germany
* Correspondence: anna-maria.kuttenreich@med.uni-jena.de; Tel.: +49-3641-9-329398

Abstract: Facial palsy is a movement disorder with impacts on verbal and nonverbal communication. The aim of this study is to investigate the effects of post-paralytic facial synkinesis on facial emotion recognition. In a prospective cross-sectional study, we compared facial emotion recognition between $n = 30$ patients with post-paralytic facial synkinesis (mean disease time: 1581 ± 1237 days) and $n = 30$ healthy controls matched in sex, age, and education level. Facial emotion recognition was measured by the *Myfacetraining* Program. As an intra-individual control condition, auditory emotion recognition was assessed via *Montreal Affective Voices*. Moreover, self-assessed emotion recognition was studied with questionnaires. In facial as well as auditory emotion recognition, on average, there was no significant difference between patients and healthy controls. The outcomes of the measurements as well as the self-reports were comparable between patients and healthy controls. In contrast to previous studies in patients with peripheral and central facial palsy, these results indicate unimpaired ability for facial emotion recognition. Only in single patients with pronounced facial asymmetry and severe facial synkinesis was an impaired facial and auditory emotion recognition detected. Further studies should compare emotion recognition in patients with pronounced facial asymmetry in acute and chronic peripheral paralysis and central and peripheral facial palsy.

Keywords: facial palsy; post-paralytic facial synkinesis; emotion recognition; facial feedback

1. Introduction

Facial palsy can affect the face in function and appearance [1] with various consequences [2]. Due to the motor impairment of the facial muscles and its effect on verbal and nonverbal communication, it can also be considered as a communication disorder [3]. Accordingly, there may be emerging constraints on verbal communication such as articulation and intelligibility [4], as well as in nonverbal communication [3]. In nonverbal communication, it can be difficult for patients with facial palsy to express facial emotions [5–8] and their conversation partners experience this impaired mimic communication [6]. The interlocutors perceive the patients' deformed appearance negatively [9], and attribute negative emotion expressions even while smiling [10]. Further, the patients are judged significantly less likeable, less trustworthy [11], and less attractive [9,11]. This external perception may lead to social exclusion [11] and stigmatisation [3,12]. About 20–30% of the

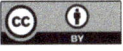

patients do not recover from facial palsy, thus continuously suffering from post-paralytic facial synkinesis [13–19], i.e., involuntary muscle movement while executing a different, intentional muscle movement [19].

Despite the fact that different negative consequences of facial palsy are already known, the communicative effects of facial palsy and post-paralytic facial synkinesis are not conclusively elucidated yet. For example, the performance of facial emotion recognition has received limited scientific attention so far, although the first indications of deficits are available in recent studies (details below) [20]. Up until today, as a review on emotion processing in patients with facial palsy summarised in the available studies, it is not finally clarified whether patients with facial palsy and especially those who suffer from post-paralytic facial synkinesis are severely and systematically affected by impaired facial emotion recognition [20].

Depending on the location of the lesion, peripheral and central facial palsy are distinguished [16]. For both types, the first evidence on facial emotion recognition is available: In a recent study, we examined the facial emotion recognition of patients with central facial paresis after a stroke. The patients demonstrated significant deficits in accuracy of facial emotion recognition when compared to patients after a stroke without facial paresis and healthy controls [21–23]. Although the results demonstrate a specific deficit in facial emotion recognition compared to auditory emotion recognition of patients with facial paresis, the cause for these limitations is not completely elucidated. Both stroke [24] and altered facial feedback [25] could influence facial emotion recognition. Consequently, facial emotion recognition should be tested in patients with altered facial feedback, e.g., with post-paralytic facial synkinesis, but without any neurological precondition [21–23].

Recent studies have also documented impaired facial emotion recognition in patients with peripheral facial palsy. For example, Storbeck et al. reported that 31 patients with acute peripheral facial palsy were significantly slower in facial emotion recognition in comparison to their healthy controls [26]. Moreover, Konnerth et al. presented similar results (significantly slower), when comparing 13 patients with chronic (>four weeks post onset) peripheral facial palsy and a healthy control group [27]. Korb et al. even identified impairments especially for patients with left-sided facial palsy [28]. However, overall, there is only a small number of studies that examine facial emotion recognition in patients with peripheral facial palsy [20].

Our present study addresses this open issue. To uncover existing deficits or competences, the aim of this study is to observe the effects of post-paralytic facial synkinesis on facial emotion recognition.

2. Materials and Methods

2.1. Study Design

In a prospective cross-sectional study, we examined patients with post-paralytic facial synkinesis and compared them to healthy controls in facial emotion recognition in accuracy and time. We also tested auditory emotion recognition to distinguish intra-individually general deficits in emotion recognition from modality-specific deficits in facial emotion recognition. Moreover, we assessed the participants' subjective judgements of their own facial emotion recognition abilities.

This selection and combination of measurements and assessments is already established and proven to be useful. It was developed in a recent study on facial emotion recognition focusing patients with central facial paresis. There, this set of measurements and assessments demonstrated reliable discrimination between patients with and without central facial paresis as well as healthy controls and uncovered deficits [21–23].

The study was conducted according to ethical standards and was approved by the ethical committee (2020-1787-BO) of the Jena University Hospital Jena, Germany. All participants signed a consent form voluntarily after they had been informed in detail about the study.

2.2. Participants

Two target groups of participants were recruited: (1) patients (adults ≥18 years) with unilateral, chronic (≥1 year post onset) peripheral facial palsy with related facial synkinesis, diagnosed by an expert physician, and (2) healthy controls (adults ≥18 years) with no history of facial palsy, and no acute or chronic facial palsy with or without facial synkinesis. All patients and healthy controls had normal or corrected vision and hearing ability assessed by the participant. None of the participants had a diagnosis of neurological or mental disorders and/or taking antidepressants.

Recruitment and data collection were conducted from 4 August 2020 to 20 August 2021. The patients were recruited at the Facial-Nerve-Center Jena, Jena University Hospital, Jena, Germany. The examinations took place either at the Jena University Hospital or during home visits if requested from the participants. None of the participants had ever received prior facial emotion recognition diagnostic or specific emotion recognition therapy.

A total of 30 patients with post-paralytic facial synkinesis and 30 healthy controls without facial palsy were included. The patients and the healthy controls were matched in pairs based on their sex, age, and education level. These three factors, sex, age, and education were selected because they may have an impact on physiological emotion recognition (sex: [29,30]; age: [31]; education level: [32]). Characteristics of the patients and the healthy controls are presented in Appendix A, Table A1. Most patients and healthy controls were female, middle aged, and with an education of medium maturity. There were no significant group differences between patients and healthy controls in sex, age and education level. Mean duration of facial palsy was 1581 ± 1237 days. Detailed information of facial palsy is provided in Appendix A, Table A2.

Diagnosis and Grading of Facial Palsy and Facial Synkinesis

In order to study the presence and grading of a possible facial palsy and facial synkinesis, all participants went through examination (conducted by a speech and language therapist) regarding facial palsy in addition to the diagnosis by a physician.

For this purpose, all participants were instructed in a standardised manner to show their face at rest and then to perform voluntary movements with their face. The examination was recorded with a video camera (CANON, HF100, Tokyo, Japan; camera at a right angle, positioned 150 cm away from the participant's chin, camera lens at the individual level of the participant's chewing plane) and graded according to the *Sunnybrook Facial Grading System* [33,34] afterwards. This tool is used to determine a composite total score (Composite Score; 0: total facial paralysis to 100: normal face) from sub scores for symmetry at rest (Resting Symmetry Score), voluntary movements (Voluntary Movement Score), and synkinesis (Synkinesis Score) [33,34]. In addition to this rating, to distinguish between faces with and without facial palsy and to ascertain the degree of facial palsy, we classified the composite total score of *Sunnybrook Facial Grading System* according the House & Brackmann *Facial Nerve Grading System* [35] into six degrees of severity: 100–84 points: normal function, no facial paresis/paralysis; 83–67: light facial paresis; 66–50 moderate facial paresis; 49–33 medium facial paresis; 32–16 severe facial paresis; 15–0 complete facial paralysis. Thus, a certain degree (16 points out of 100 points) of asymmetry was accepted as physiological.

Facial palsy was excluded in all healthy controls (Composite Score: Mean = 91.3 ± 4.5; Grade Median = 1). In all patients, facial synkinesis was confirmed (Composite Score: Mean = 39.4 ± 15.8). About half of the patients had medium facial paresis (Grade Median = 4). Abnormalities were observed in all patients through resting symmetry (Resting Symmetry Score: Median = 15), voluntary movement (Voluntary Movement Score: Median = 58), and synkinesis (Synkinesis Score: Median = 6). Thus, all patients had unilateral facial synkinesis [15–17,19]. About half of the patients were affected on the left side, while the other half of the patients were affected on the right side of their face. Detailed information on the diagnosis, affected side, grading, aetiology, and the time post onset of the facial palsy (patients), or facial integrity (healthy controls) can be found in Appendix A, Table A2.

2.3. Materials for Measuring Facial and Auditory Emotion Recognition and Self-Assessment of Facial Emotion Recognition

In order to test emotion recognition, the so-called basic emotions of anger, disgust, fear, joy, sadness, and surprise [36,37] were used. These emotions are considered as unambiguous and culture-independent [38] and are typically used for this purpose [39].

We examined all participants once. For measuring emotion recognition, the accuracy (percentage of correctly recognised items) and time (average speed in seconds) were recorded in facial and auditory modality. To ensure that the tasks were understood by the participants, a pre-test with ten items was presented beforehand. These procedures are explained in the following sections and has already been established and described in more detail before [21–23].

2.3.1. Measuring Facial Emotion Recognition

Data of facial emotion recognition was collected using the *Myfacetraining* (MFT) Program (CRAFTA Cranio Facial Therapy Academy, Hamburg, Germany; [40,41]). Each participant rated 42 photographs of people showing one of the six basic emotions on their face. The participants were asked to choose the presented emotion from different options within ten seconds as correctly and quickly as possible (presented from a laptop Lenovo yoga 500 (Lenovo, Hongkong, China), screen size 14 inches, touch screen input mode) see also [21–23].

2.3.2. Measuring Auditory Emotion Recognition

To test auditory emotion recognition, a selection (basic emotions) of the *Montreal Affective Voices* (MAV) [42] was presented. The participants were asked to rate a total number of 60 emotional, non-linguistic, vocal expressions (on/a:/) of the basic emotions by selecting the presented emotion from different options as correctly and quickly as possible. Each item was presented once and ten seconds responding time was given (input mode: point on symbols on a DIN-A4 paper sheet) through a specially programmed experiment in PsychoPy (version 3.0.0b9; [43]; laptop Lenovo yoga 500 (Lenovo, Hongkong, China), screen size 14 inches, using commercially available wired headband headphones with an individual volume at the participant's discretion), see also [21–23].

2.3.3. Self-Assessment of Facial Emotion Recognition

To self-assess facial emotion recognition, all participants filled out four questionnaires for two categories:

(1) *Overall competence in accuracy and time:* Two questionnaires were developed to assess overall competence in facial emotion recognition on a visual analogue scale (10 cm). All participants were asked how accurate (questionnaire for accuracy) and how fast (questionnaire for time) they would rate themselves in recognising the six basic emotions in other people's faces.
(2) *Changes in accuracy and time since facial palsy:* Further, we adapted and used two questionnaires (one for accuracy, one for time) [21–23] to assess possible changes in facial emotion recognition since the onset of their facial palsy. The patients were asked whether they noticed changes in accuracy and time, when recognising each of the six basic emotions in other faces (−1 point: less accurate/slower; 0 points: no change; +1 point: more accurate/faster). Moreover, the healthy controls were requested if they noticed any changes over a comparable period of time (average time of facial palsy duration in patients: mean = 1581 days ≙ 4 years; see also Appendix A, Table A2).

2.4. Statistical Analysis

All data were analysed using Microsoft Excel 2019 (Redmond, WA, USA; [44] and IBM SPSS Statistics 28.0 (Armonk, NY, USA; [45]. Results at an alpha level of $p < 0.05$ were considered significant.

To compare the results of facial and auditory emotion recognition (accuracy and time) obtained from the patients and the healthy controls, 2 × 2 ANOVAs with *group* (patients vs. healthy controls) as between-subject factor and *modality* (facial vs. auditory) as within-subject repeated-measures factor were conducted. Significant interactions were resolved by post hoc *t*-tests for dependent samples to test facial vs. auditory emotion recognition (accuracy and time) separately within each group of participants.

In addition to this analysis of emotion recognition, factors were explored, which are systematically related to the performance of emotion recognition. If such factors could be identified, they may provide further insight on emotion recognition and could be considered in the evidence-based care of patients with facial palsy. Therefore, correlations for facial and auditory emotion recognition in accuracy and time (Pearson) as well as accuracy/time and sex (Pearson), age (Pearson), education (Spearman), overall severity of facial palsy (Pearson), and separately sub scores resting symmetry, voluntary movements, and facial synkinesis (Spearman) were calculated. Moreover, *t*-tests for independent samples to test the facial emotion recognition of patients with left- and right-sided facial synkinesis were run.

In a last step, the self-assessment of the patients and the healthy controls in emotion recognition (accuracy and time) were compared through *t*-tests for independent samples, and within each group of participants (patients or healthy controls) through *t*-tests for dependent samples. Moreover, correlations for self-assessed facial emotion recognition in accuracy and time (Pearson) as well as self-assessed and measured facial emotion recognition (Pearson) were conducted.

3. Results

The results of measured facial and auditory emotion recognition as well as computed ANOVAs and *t*-tests are presented separately by accuracy and time. Significant results are reported in text and all results (significant and not significant) are summarised in Table 1. In further analysis, announced correlations are reported. Finally, the results for self-assessment and its correlations are described.

Table 1. Results of measured facial emotion recognition (FER)-accuracy/time, and auditory emotion recognition (AER)-accuracy/time.

Measured Emotion Recognition	Patients $n = 30$	Healthy Controls $n = 30$
	Mean ± SD Min, Max	Mean ± SD Min, Max
FER Accuracy via MFT Program in %	67.7 ± 11.3 Min 29 Max 86	69.1 ± 9.2 Min 48 Max 86
FER Time via MFT Program in seconds	4.2 ± 0.8 Min 2.6 Max 6.4	4.2 ± 0.6 Min 3.2 Max 5.8
AER Accuracy via MAV in %	64.9 ± 11.3 Min 25 Max 83.3	65.6 ± 10.3 Min 45 Max 80
AER Time via MAV in seconds	2.7 ± 0.6 Min 1.9 Max 5	2.8 ± 0.7 Min 1.8 Max 5

Table 1. Cont.

Statistical analysis	Main effect of modality	Main effect of group	Interaction effect of modality × group
	2 × 2 ANOVA p	2 × 2 ANOVA p	2 × 2 ANOVA p
Accuracy	$F(1; 58) = 7.387$ $p = 0.009$	$F(1; 58) = 0.170$ $p = 0.682$	$F(1; 58) = 0.093$ $p = 0.762$
Time	$F(1; 58) = 441.501$ $p < 0.001$	$F(1; 58) = 0.170$ $p = 0.682$	$F(1; 58) = 0.219$ $p = 0.641$

3.1. Accuracy

The 2 × 2 ANOVA yielded a significant main effect of *modality*, with higher accuracy in facial emotion recognition than in auditory emotion recognition.

No significant main effect of *group*, and no significant interaction effect of *group × modality* was identified.

Table 1 shows the results of measured emotion recognition and the statistical analysis. Figure 1 shows facial and auditory emotion recognition in accuracy as a function of time post onset.

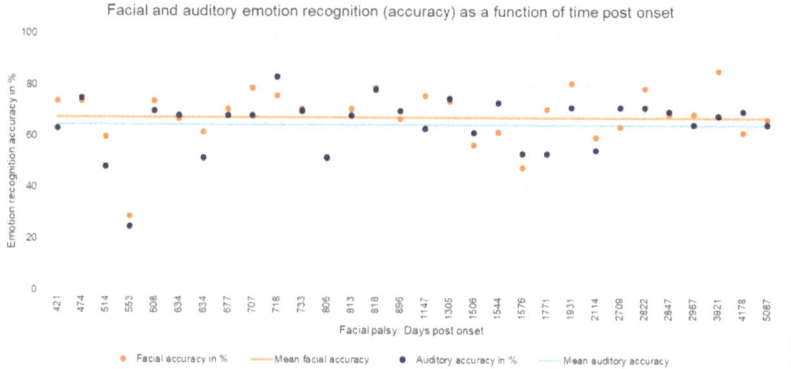

Figure 1. Facial and auditory emotion recognition (accuracy) as a function of time post onset. Individual results of the patients with facial synkinesis are shown as dots in bright orange (facial accuracy) and bright blue (auditory accuracy). Mean of facial accuracy in the patient group is shown as a line in pastel orange, and mean of auditory accuracy in the patient group is shown as a line in pastel blue.

3.2. Time

The 2 × 2 ANOVA yielded a significant main effect of *modality*, with longer response times in facial emotion recognition than in auditory emotion recognition.

No significant main effect of *group*, and no significant interaction effect of *group × modality* was identified.

Table 1 shows the results of measured emotion recognition and the statistical analysis. Figure 2 shows the facial and auditory emotion recognition in time as a function of time post onset.

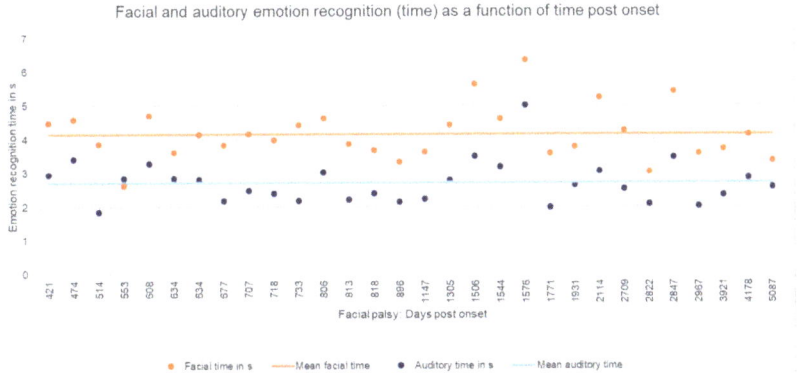

Figure 2. Facial and auditory emotion recognition (time) as a function of time post onset. Individual results of the patients with facial synkinesis are shown as dots in bright orange (facial time) and bright blue (auditory time). Mean of facial accuracy in the patient group is shown as line in pastel orange, and mean of auditory accuracy in the patient group is shown as a line in pastel blue.

Table 1 shows an overview of all results of the measured emotion recognition. No significant differences were found between patients and healthy controls, but within each participant group, depending on the tested modality.

3.3. Further Analysis of Measured Facial Emotion Recognition

For further analysis, we studied different possible correlations as described in the section of *Statistical Analysis*. All results in correlations (significant and not significant) are summarised in Tables 2–4. Significant correlations are also presented in the text.

Table 2. Correlations between facial emotion recognition (FER)-accuracy/time, and auditory emotion recognition (AER)-accuracy/time.

Correlations	FER Accuracy		FER Time	
	Pearson r	p	Pearson r	p
FER Time				
All participants	−0.150	0.126		
Patients	−0.167	0.189		
Healthy controls	−0.131	0.245		
AER Accuracy				
All participants	**0.650**	**<0.001**		
Patients	**0.781**	**<0.001**		
Healthy controls	**0.473**	**0.004**		
AER Time				
All participants			**0.712**	**<0.001**
Patients			**0.788**	**<0.001**
Healthy controls			**0.638**	**<0.001**

Significant correlations are marked bold.

Table 3. Correlations between facial emotion recognition (FER)-accuracy/time, and sex, age, and education.

Correlations	FER Accuracy		FER Time	
	Pearson r	p	Pearson r	p
Sex				
All participants	**−0.220**	**0.046**	0.134	0.153
Patients	−0.221	0.121	0.187	0.161
Healthy controls	−0.222	0.119	0.071	0.356
Age				
All participants	**−0.427**	**<0.001**	**0.339**	**0.004**
Patients	**−0.398**	**0.015**	**0.340**	**0.033**
Healthy controls	**−0.468**	**0.005**	**0.345**	**0.031**
	Spearman ρ	p	Spearman ρ	p
Education				
All participants	**0.291**	**0.012**	−0.067	0.304
Patients	0.213	0.129	−0.029	0.440
Healthy controls	**0.367**	**0.023**	−0.102	0.296

Significant correlations are marked bold.

Table 4. Correlations between facial emotion recognition (FER)-accuracy/time, and auditory emotion recognition (AER)-accuracy/time, and resting facial symmetry, and facial synkinesis.

Correlations	FER Accuracy	FER Time	AER Accuracy	AER Time
	Pearson r / p	Pearson r / p	Pearson r / p	Pearson r / p
Composite Score				
All participants	0.127 / 0.168	−0.062 / 0.320	0.072 / 0.293	−0.032 / 0.405
	Spearman ρ / p	Spearman ρ / p	Spearman ρ / p	Spearman ρ / p
Resting Symmetry Score				
Patients	**−0.441 / 0.007**	0.051 / 0.304	−0.103 / 0.295	0.187 / 0.161
Healthy controls	0.163 / 0.195	0.151 / 0.213	0.096 / 0.307	0.120 / 0.264
Resting Symmetry Eye				
Patients	−0.240 / 0.100	0.093 / 0.313	−0.124 / 0.257	0.108 / 0.285
Healthy controls	0.265 / 0.079	−0.041 / 0.414	0.166 / 0.190	0.274 / 0.072
Resting Symmetry Cheek				
Patients	−0.041 / 0.414	0.181 / 0.169	−0.218 / 0.123	0.062 / 0.372
Healthy controls	0.076 / 0.344	0.084 / 0.330	0.124 / 0.256	−0.148 / 0.218

Table 4. Cont.

	Spearman ρ p	Spearman ρ p	Spearman ρ p	Spearman ρ p
Resting Symmetry Mouth				
Patients	**−0.353** **0.028**	0.087 0.324	−0.058 0.380	0.029 0.440
Healthy controls	−0.106 0.288	0.164 0.194	−0.184 0.166	0.091 0.315
Voluntary Movement Score				
Patients	−0.013 0.473	−0.139 0.232	−0.079 0.338	−0.165 0.192
Healthy controls	0.223 0.118	−0.166 0.190	0.205 0.138	−0.048 0.400
Synkinesis Score				
Patients	**−0.348** **0.030**	0.267 0.077	**−0.474** **0.004**	**0.334** **0.035**
Synkinesis in Brow lift				
Patients	−0.234 0.107	0.038 0.421	−0.295 0.057	0.093 0.313
Synkinesis in Gentle eye closure				
Patients	0.071 0.355	−0.210 0.133	**−0.383** **0.018**	0.020 0.457
Synkinesis in Open mouth smile				
Patients	−0.298 0.055	0.263 0.080	**−0.326** **0.040**	0.267 0.077
Synkinesis in Snarl				
Patients	**−0.334** **0.036**	**0.441** **0.007**	−0.244 0.097	**0.394** **0.016**
Synkinesis in Lip pucker				
Patients	−0.218 0.124	0.221 0.120	**−0.484** **0.003**	0.227 0.114

Significant correlations are marked bold.

3.3.1. Correlation between Accuracy and Time in Measured Facial and Auditory Emotion Recognition

There was a significant positive correlation between accuracy for facial emotion recognition and accuracy for auditory emotion recognition for all participants as well as in the patients, and in the healthy controls.

There was a significant negative correlation between accuracy for facial emotion recognition and time for auditory emotion recognition for all participants, and in the patients.

There was a significant negative correlation between time for facial emotion recognition and accuracy for auditory emotion recognition in the healthy controls.

There was a significant positive correlation between time for facial emotion recognition and time for auditory emotion recognition for all participants as well as in the patients, and in the healthy controls.

3.3.2. Correlation between Accuracy/Time of Measured Facial Emotion Recognition and Sex

There was a significant negative correlation between accuracy and sex across all participants, with higher accuracy for females.

3.3.3. Correlation between Accuracy/Time of Measured Facial Emotion Recognition and Age

There was a significant negative correlation between accuracy and age across all participants (Figure 3).

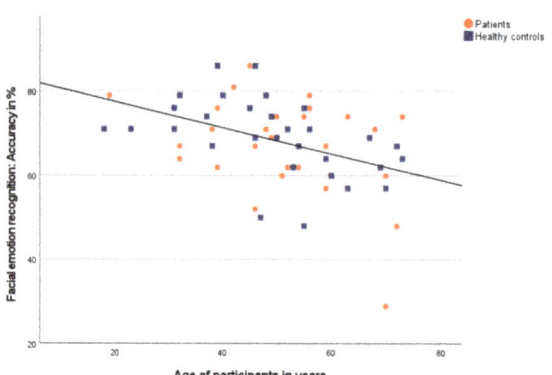

Figure 3. Correlation between accuracy of facial emotion recognition and age. Patients are shown as orange dots, and healthy controls as blue squares.

There was a significant positive correlation between time and age across all participants (Figure 4).

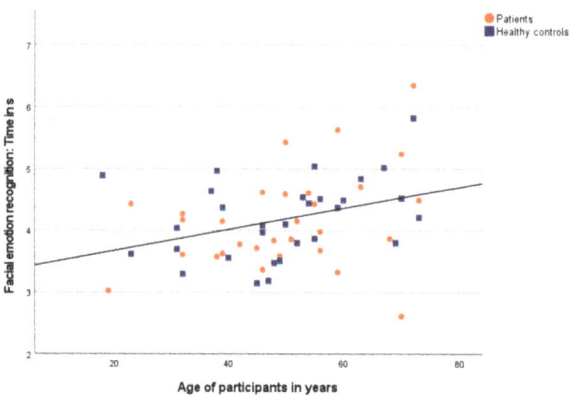

Figure 4. Correlation between time of facial emotion recognition and age. Patients are shown as orange dots, and healthy controls as blue squares.

Further, when examining the patients, there was a significant negative correlation between accuracy and age as well as a significant positive correlation between time and age. Similarly, the measures of the healthy controls correlated significantly negative between accuracy and age as well as significantly positive between time and age.

3.3.4. Correlation between Accuracy/Time of Measured Facial Emotion Recognition and Education

There was a significant positive correlation between accuracy and education across all participants. The measures of the healthy controls demonstrated a significant positive correlation between accuracy and education.

3.3.5. Correlation between Accuracy/Time of Measured Facial Emotion Recognition and Overall Grading of Facial Palsy

Figures 5 and 6 show correlations between accuracy/time of measured facial emotion recognition and overall grading of facial palsy *(Sunnybrook Facial Grading System: Composite Score).*

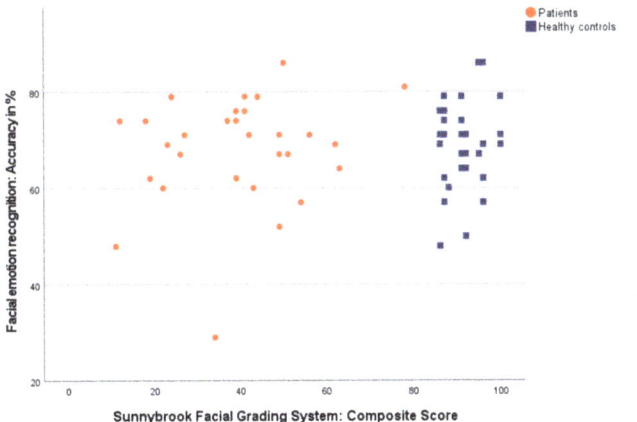

Figure 5. Correlation between accuracy of facial emotion recognition and grading of facial palsy. Patients are shown as orange dots, and healthy controls as blue squares.

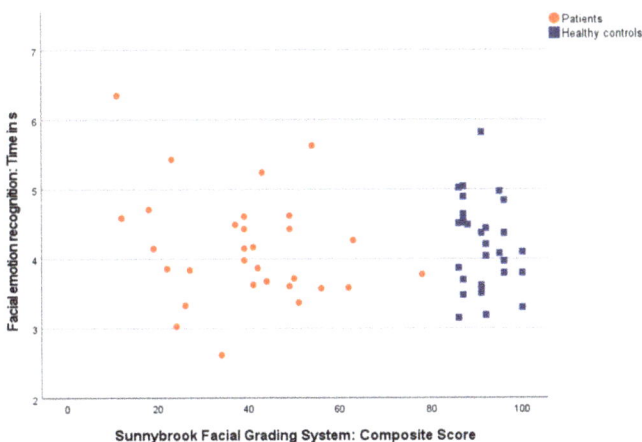

Figure 6. Correlation between time of facial emotion recognition and grading of facial palsy. Patients are shown as orange dots, and healthy controls as blue squares.

3.3.6. Correlation between Accuracy/Time of Measured Facial and Auditory Emotion Recognition and Facial Resting Symmetry

In the patients, there was a significant negative correlation between accuracy for facial emotion recognition and facial resting symmetry *(Sunnybrook Facial Grading System: Resting*

Symmetry Score). Moreover, in patients, there was a significant negative correlation between accuracy for facial emotion recognition and resting symmetry mouth.

3.3.7. Correlation between Accuracy/Time of Measured Facial and Auditory Emotion Recognition and Facial Synkinesis

In the patients, there were significant negative correlations between accuracy for facial emotion recognition and facial synkinesis *(Sunnybrook Facial Grading System: Synkinesis Score)* and synkinesis in snarl. Moreover, in patients, there was a significant positive correlation between time for facial emotion recognition and synkinesis in snarl.

In the patients, there was a significant negative correlation between accuracy for auditory emotion recognition and facial synkinesis *(Sunnybrook Facial Grading System: Synkinesis Score)*. Moreover, in patients, there were significant negative correlations between accuracy for auditory emotion recognition and synkinesis of gentle eye closure, open mouth smile, and lip pucker. In the patients, there was a significant positive correlation between time for auditory emotion recognition and facial synkinesis (Sunnybrook Facial Grading System: Synkinesis Score). Moreover, in patients, there was a significant positive correlation between time for auditory emotion recognition and synkinesis in snarl.

3.3.8. Accuracy/Time of Measured Facial Emotion recognition and Affected Side of Facial Synkinesis

Further, we performed *t*-tests to compare the facial emotion recognition of patients with left- and right-sided facial synkinesis.

A one-tailed *t*-test for independent samples for facial emotion recognition showed a trend for significance in accuracy between the patients with left-sided (Mean = 70.88 ± 8.25) and the patients with right-sided (Mean = 64.07 ± 13.45) facial synkinesis, t(28) = 1.694; *p* = 0.051.

A one-tailed *t*-test for independent samples for facial emotion recognition demonstrated no significant difference in time between the patients with left-sided (Mean = 4.15 ± 0.54) and the patients with right-sided (Mean = 4.22 ± 1.02) facial synkinesis, t(28) = −0.398; *p* = 0.347.

3.4. Self-Assessing Facial Emotion Recognition

Table 5 shows all the results of the self-assessed facial emotion recognition.

Table 5. Results of self-assessed facial emotion recognition (accuracy and time).

Facial Emotion Recognition: Self-Assessment Questionnaire	Patients $n = 30$	Healthy Controls $n = 30$
	Mean ± SD Min, Max	Mean ± SD Min, Max
Overall competence: Accuracy	43.4 ± 7.5 Min 22.6 Max 54.4	43.8 ± 5.9 Min 26.1 Max 51.9
Overall competence: Time	41.7 ± 8.7 Min 16.7 Max 53.4	40.5 ± 8.9 Min 19.6 Max 53.5
Changes: Accuracy	0.1 ± 1.6 Min −4 Max 6	0.5 ± 1.1 Min −2 Max 3
Changes: Time	−0.2 ± 2.1 Min −6 Max 6	−0.1 ± 2.3 Min −6 Max 5

3.4.1. Overall Competence

The *t*-test examining accuracy demonstrated no significant difference between the patients and the healthy controls, t(58) = −2.38; p = 0.406. Moreover, the *t*-test examining time demonstrated no significant difference between the patients and the healthy controls, t(58) = 0.523; p = 0.302.

The *t*-tests within the groups demonstrated a significant higher self-assessment in accuracy, in comparison to time for the patients, t(29) = 1.894; p = 0.034. The same results go for the healthy controls, with a significant higher self-assessment in accuracy, in comparison to time, t(29) = 2.658; p = 0.006.

3.4.2. Changes since Facial Palsy

The *t*-test examining accuracy demonstrated no significant difference between the patients and the healthy controls, t(58) = −1.134; p = 0.131. Moreover, the *t*-test examining time demonstrated no significant difference between the patients and the healthy controls, t(58) = −0.179; p = 0.429.

The *t*-test within the groups demonstrated no significant difference in accuracy, in comparison to time for the patients, t(29) = 1.179; p = 0.124. The same results go for the healthy controls with no significant difference in accuracy, in comparison to time, t(29) = 1.582; p = 0.062.

3.4.3. Correlation between Accuracy and Time in Self-Assessed Facial Emotion Recognition

There was a significant correlation between self-assessed accuracy and time for facial emotion recognition in the patients, r = 0.829 (p < 0.001), and in the healthy controls, r = 0.653 (p < 0.001).

3.4.4. Correlation between Accuracy and Time in Self-Assessed and Measured Facial Emotion Recognition

In the healthy controls, there was a significant correlation between self-assessed accuracy and measured accuracy for facial emotion recognition.

In the healthy controls, there was a significant correlation between self-assessed time and measured accuracy for facial emotion recognition (Table 6).

Table 6. Correlations between measured and self-assessed facial emotion recognition (FER)-accuracy/time.

Correlations	Measured FER Accuracy		Measured FER Time	
	Pearson r	p	Pearson r	p
Self-assessed FER Accuracy				
Patients	0.182	0.168	0.201	0.144
Healthy controls	**0.438**	**0.008**	−0.090	0.318
Self-assessed FER Time				
Patients	0.268	0.076	0.196	0.150
Healthy controls	**0.381**	**0.019**	−0.030	0.438

Significant correlations are marked bold.

4. Discussion

The aim of this study is to observe the effects of post-paralytic facial synkinesis on facial emotion recognition. For this purpose, we examined patients with facial synkinesis and healthy controls in facial and auditory emotion recognition. The results of the standardised measurements as well as the self-reports present similar outcomes on facial and auditory emotion recognition between the groups of patients and healthy controls. Only in single cases, there were impairments, i.e., only limited performance, in facial and auditory emotion recognition in patients with pronounced facial asymmetry and facial synkinesis. Consequently, facial emotion recognition is a present competence of patients with facial synkinesis. The results will presently be discussed in more detail.

4.1. Comparison with Other Studies of Emotion Recognition and Facial Palsy

In a pilot study, Konnerth et al. [27], examined $n = 13$ patients with chronic peripheral facial palsy (sex: female 53.80%, male 46.20%; age: mean = 53.00 ± 17.64 years; facial palsy duration: mean = 7.82 ± 15.00 years). Facial emotion recognition resulted in average accuracy of 76.71 ± 12.60% and average time of 2.89 ± 0.95 s. By contrast, the patients in our study demonstrated lower accuracy and longer reaction times.

Storbeck et al. [26] studied $n = 31$ patients with acute peripheral facial palsy (sex: female 41.94%, male 58.06%; age: mean = 40.00 ± 2.3 years; facial palsy duration: mean = 7 ± 0.7 days and average moderate to moderately serve facial palsy). The facial emotion recognition resulted in an accuracy of 68.15 ± 2.25% and time of 10.77 ± 0.84 s (average data for test point t1). All the patients of our study demonstrated nearly similar performances in accuracy, but higher performance in time.

For both previous studies, an ideal comparison with our study in facial emotion recognition cannot be conducted, because of the difference in the examination procedure and the sample compositions. Even so, since there are only a small number of studies examine emotion recognition in patients with facial palsy, the results should be considered [20]. Both studies used different emotion recognition tasks, whereby Konnerth et al. [27] is quite closer to the tools, used by us. The sex and age distribution differs as well as the time post onset facial palsy and its grading. Besides this incomparability between the studies, these may be factors that led to identification of deficits in facial emotion recognition time in contrast to healthy controls. In our study, we cannot confirm deficits in accuracy and time, but measured unimpaired facial and auditory emotion recognition. In future studies, facial emotion recognition should be tested with the same tool (1) at patients with acute and chronic facial palsy. This will make the results for different time stages post onset facial palsy comparable. It could be that facial emotion recognition is impaired in the early stage of acute facial palsy and recovers or could compensate in the chronic phase. In such an analysis, the typical course (paralytic, paretic, and possible synkinesis) [16,18] of facial palsy should be considered. Further on, (2) patients with acute and chronic flaccid paralysis with pronounced asymmetry should also be taken into account. Thus, the impact of facial asymmetry on facial emotion recognition can be investigated to a greater extent.

4.2. Emotion Recognition Depending on Facial Palsy

In line with Storbeck et al. (2019), our results reached the same conclusion regarding the correlation of facial emotion recognition and facial palsy. Storbeck et al. described no correlation between accuracy as well as time in facial emotion recognition and an overall grading of facial palsy [26], and neither did we. In total, this suggests the subordinate impact of facial feedback on facial emotion recognition. In particular, unilateral facial synkinesis, which may result in altered facial feedback, did not interrupt facial emotion recognition at first sight. But a detailed consideration of facial palsy provides new insights.

In contrast to Storbeck et al. (2019), who used the global *Facial Nerve Grading System 2.0* [46], we chose the comparatively finer-grained *Sunnybrook Facial Grading System* [33,34] for facial palsy grading. The separate assessment of resting symmetry, voluntary movements, and synkinesis in the *Sunnybrook Facial Grading System* [33,34] enables one to determine the significant correlation factors of asymmetry and synkinesis on facial and auditory emotion recognition in patients. The more asymmetric the face at rest, the less accurate was the measured facial emotion recognition. The more facial synkinesis, the less accurate and slower was the measured facial and auditory emotion recognition. For this, facial asymmetry may compromise individual patients in single cases in their accuracy of facial emotion recognition, especially for asymmetry in the mouth. Synkinesis may compromise patients' facial and auditory accuracy and response time, especially for synkinesis in voluntary gentle eye closure, open mouth smile, snarl, and lip pucker.

Synkinesis can lead to altered facial feedback, such as the so-called *autoparalytic syndrome*, in which different facial muscles interfere and inhibit each other [19]. The correlation between synkinesis and facial emotion recognition can be obviously explained by the facial feedback hypothesis, in which facial feedback is essential for successful facial emotion recognition [25]. While the correlation between synkinesis and auditory emotion recognition may be surprising at first, the effect of altered facial feedback in auditory emotion recognition is in line with previous research. Coles et al. (2019) cleared in their meta-analysis the significant effect of facial feedback and its dependence on the type of stimulus. While visual stimuli demonstrated a small effect, auditory stimuli was pointed out with high effects [47]. Thus, auditory emotion recognition can be affected by altered facial feedback [48]. Such as in prior research [48,49], our results may support evidence for facial feedback in overall emotion processing, and not only in facial emotion recognition, but also in auditory emotion recognition. In our sample, required facial feedback was still partially presented, e.g., because of unilateral (not bilateral) facial palsy. But in individual cases that particularly serve impairments in asymmetry and synkinesis, the facial feedback seemed to no longer be sufficient, and facial as well as auditory emotion recognition becomes affected.

Related to the side of the face, Korb et al. [28] reported an advantage in facial emotion recognition of patients with facial palsy on the right side in comparison to patients with facial palsy on the left side. We stated no significant difference in facial emotion recognition between patients with left- and right-sided facial synkinesis. However, in our data, there was a strong trend for a reversed effect. This aspect will thus need further attention in future research.

4.3. Comparison with Other Studies of Facial and Auditory Emotion Recognition

To test both facial and auditory emotion recognition within one study is rare in the previous literature [50]. Existing evidence demonstrates higher performance in facial than auditory emotion recognition [51–53]. In our study, the patients as well as the healthy controls were significantly more accurate but significantly slower in facial emotion recognition in comparison to auditory emotion recognition. Therefore, our results confirm existing evidence in accuracy while providing new evidence for a contrast in facial and auditory emotion recognition. For our sample (both patients and healthy controls), the statistical analysis revealed systematic significant correlations between facial and auditory emotion recognition. The more accurate the facial emotion recognition, the more accurate the auditory emotion recognition. The faster the facial emotion recognition, the faster the auditory emotion recognition. Thus, the ability to recognise emotions, regardless of modality, is more or less powerful within a person.

4.4. Correlations for Facial Emotion Recognition on Sex, Age, and Education

Additional factors demonstrated significant correlations on measured facial emotion recognition.

Among all participants, a correlation between accuracy and sex was noticeable. Women detected facially expressed emotions more accurately than men. These findings are consistent with previous research [29,30].

For all participants, the accuracy correlated significantly negative and the time correlated significantly positive with age. That means with increasing age, accuracy in facial emotion recognition decreased while time rises. Moreover, these results are in agreement with previous findings [31].

For all participants, there was a correlation between accuracy and education. This means, participants with higher education were more accurate in facial emotion recognition. Again, these findings are in line with previous research [32].

4.5. Self-Assessed Facial Emotion Recognition

We recorded self-assessed facial emotion recognition standardised in all participants. The more accurately participants (patients and healthy controls) assessed themselves in facial emotion recognition, the faster they assessed themselves. But only in the healthy controls, the more accurately and faster healthy controls assessed themselves in facial emotion recognition, the more accurate was the measured facial emotion recognition. This systematic significant correlation did not exist in patients. Thus, the patients' self-assessment was less adequate compared to the measured emotion recognition.

4.6. Quality of Diagnostic Instruments

With our presented assessment of facial emotion recognition (cf. [21–23], we tested facial emotion recognition of patients with facial synkinesis. To construct different control parameters, we examined healthy controls without facial palsy and auditory emotion recognition as well.

While we have uncovered impaired facial emotion recognition (accuracy) in patients with central facial palsy before [21–23], we revealed results regarding the abilities of patients with facial synkinesis. Besides the measurements, we took into consideration the participants' perspective with established (cf. [21–23], and newly developed questionnaires. Through the suggested measurement and self-assessment, we differentiated the participants (patients and healthy controls) and the patient groups (central and peripheral facial palsy) and detected deficits and competences. We also replicated expected correlation factors such as sex, age, and education, and new correlation factors such as asymmetry, facial synkinesis, and self-assessment, which further validates the quality of used diagnostic instruments.

4.7. Limitations of the Study

Emotions are usually not unimodal (facial or auditory), but multimodal [54]. A separation seems to be artificial, but enables us to declare the impact of facial feedback on facial emotion recognition. Since in this study the patients and healthy controls demonstrated no significant differences in facial emotion recognition, altered facial feedback (1) does not appear to have decisive influence or (2) is compensated already, where compensation by other modalities or context is excluded in this study design.

Furthermore, we solely tested basic emotions. In everyday life, more complex [38] and combinate [55] emotions have to be recognised in communication. Taking this perspective into consideration, the selection of basic emotions seems to be too experimental and unsuitable for everyday life. Further, the task of recognising basic emotions was maybe too basal, and deficits would become apparent in more complex and dynamic structures [56]. Or, it is the opposite and the stimuli were too obvious, and deficits in emotion recognition would even appear in slighter emotion expressions [49]. However, the choice of basic emotions is recommended [39] and that allows comparison with previous studies of patients with peripheral facial palsy (see above). Prospectively, performances of patients with central facial palsy should also be compared to reveal differences and parallels. After this research issue, the examination of facial emotion recognition should be improved through the expansion of multimodal and contextual information. Further studies should use more dynamic items and a variety of complex and combined emotions (c.f. [57,58]). All participants were examined, standardized via the *Sunnybrook Facial Grading System* [33,34], to rate their face (rest position, voluntary movements, and facial synkinesis) by a speech and language therapist. In future research, grading could be improved by machine learning approaches using facial landmarks [59–62] to be observer-independent [63]. An automatic assessment is of scientific value, because facial palsy and facial synkinesis as well as distinction between patients and healthy controls will become more standardised, objectified and thus more valid, reliable, and comparable within our study, and with other studies [60–62,64].

4.8. Consequences for the Care of Patients with Facial Synkinesis in Speech and Language Therapy

Up until now, high quality evidence in speech and language therapy for patients with facial palsy is rare but needed [65]. For evidence-based management, first, the impact of facial palsy and its consequences, such as facial synkinesis, have to be identified and described.

Our study introduced present competences in facial emotion recognition and call attention to the now uncovered risk of limitations in single cases of patients with pronounced facial asymmetry, and facial synkinesis as well as partially inadequate self-assessment.

According to our results, the face of patients with facial palsy should be evaluated as a part of the standard clinical routine, for example by a speech and language therapist. In individual cases with pronounced facial asymmetry and serve facial synkinesis, facial and auditory emotion recognition should be quantified via objective measurements as well as with self-assessments of facial and auditory emotion recognition. Exclusively recording of self-assessment is not sufficient, as it may be inadequate. Any limitations indicate that therapy for emotion recognition is needed and should be offered. Next to speech and language therapy, psychology should be consulted as well. If there are no limitations but intact ability, facial emotion recognition should be considered as a resource of patients with facial synkinesis. The ability to understand facial emotion expressions may support the already affected verbal and nonverbal communication of these patients and their conversation partners. The intact facial emotion recognition should be integrated and strengthened in speech and language therapy.

5. Conclusions

Facial emotion recognition is a present competence of patients with post-paralytic facial synkinesis. This resource should be integrated and strengthened in facial therapy. In future studies, the performance in the facial emotion recognition of patients with pronounced facial asymmetry in facial paralysis as well as central and peripheral facial palsy should be compared with objective instrument-based and also with standardised self-assessment tools in order to reveal differences and parallels.

Author Contributions: Conceptualization: A.-M.K., G.F.V. and S.H.; methodology: A.-M.K., G.F.V. and S.H.; software: A.-M.K.; validation: A.-M.K.; formal analysis: A.-M.K.; investigation: A.-M.K.; resources: A.-M.K., G.F.V., O.G.-L., H.v.P. and S.H.; data curation: A.-M.K.; writing—original draft preparation: A.-M.K.; writing—review and editing: A.-M.K., G.F.V., O.G.-L., H.v.P. and S.H.; visualization: A.-M.K.; supervision: G.F.V. and S.H.; project administration: A.-M.K.; funding acquisition: G.F.V. and O.G.-L. All authors have read and agreed to the published version of the manuscript.

Funding: Orlando Guntinas-Lichius was funded by the German Research Foundation (DFG, GU-463-12-1). The APC was funded by Thüringer Universitäts- und Landesbibliothek Jena.

Institutional Review Board Statement: All subjects gave their informed consent for inclusion before they participated in the study. The study was conducted according to the guidelines of the Declaration of Helsinki, and approved by the Ethics Committee of Jena University Hospital, Germany (protocol code 2020-1787-BO, 3 June 2020).

Informed Consent Statement: Informed consent was obtained from all subjects involved in the study.

Data Availability Statement: The data presented in this study are available on request from the corresponding author. The data are not publicly available due to the data being collected within a large research project that has not yet been completed.

Conflicts of Interest: The authors declare no conflict of interest.

Appendix A

Table A1. Sociodemographic information about sex, age, and education of participants.

Sociodemographic Information	Patients n = 30		Healthy Controls n = 30		Statistical Analysis
	n	%	n	%	Test p
Sex Female Male	22 8	73.3 26.7	22 8	73.3 26.7	Chi-square test $Chi^2(1) = 0.000$ $p = 1.000$
Education No certificate of education Sec. School certificate Medium maturity High school	0 4 15 11	13.3 50.0 36.7	0 4 15 11	13.3 50.0 36.7	Median test $M(1) = 0.072$ $p = 0.789$
	Mean ± SD Min, Max		Mean ± SD Min, Max		
Age in years	49.6 ± 14.1 Min 19 Max 73		49.3 ± 14.3 Min 18 Max 73		Two-tailed t-test for independent samples $t(58) = 0.091$ $p = 0.928$

Table A2. Information on facial palsy and facial integrity.

Facial Palsy vs. Facial Integrity	Patients n = 30		Healthy Controls n = 30		Statistical Analysis
	n	%	n	%	Test p
Diagnosis of facial palsy	30	100			Chi-square test $Chi^2(1) = 0.000$ $p = 1.000$
Affected side Left Right	16 14	53.3 46.7			Chi-square test $Chi^2(1) = 0.133$ $p = 0.715$
	Median Min, Max		Median Min, Max		Test p
Sunnybrook Facial Grading System					
Resting Symmetry Score (0–20)	15 Min 5 Max 15		5 Min 0 Max 10		Median test $M(1) = 27.075$ $p < 0.001$
Voluntary Movement Score (0–100)	58 Min 36 Max 88		96 Min 88 Max 100		$M(1) = 53.325$ $p < 0.001$
Synkinesis Score (0–15)	6 Min 2 Max 14		0 Min 0 Max 0		$M(1) = 56.067$ $p < 0.001$

Table A2. Cont.

	Mean ± SD Min, Max	Mean ± SD Min, Max	Test p
Sunnybrook Facial Grading System Composite Score (0–100)	39.4 ± 15.8 Min 11 Max 78	91.3 ± 4.5 Min 86 Max 100	t-test for independent samples t(33.767) = 17.308 p < 0.001
	Median Min, Max	Median Min, Max	Test p
Grading according to House & Brackmann Facial Nerve Grading System	4 Min 2 Max 6	1 Min 1 Max 1	Median test M(1) = 56.067 p < 0.001
	n %	n %	Test p
Grading according to House & Brackmann Facial Nerve Grading System Grade I Grade II Grade III Grade IV Grade V Grade VI	 0 0 1 3.3 6 20 14 46.7 7 23.3 2 6.7	 30 100 	Chi-square test Chi²(1) = 0.000 p = 1.000
Etiology Idiopathic Infectious/inflammatory Iatrogenic Neoplastic	 16 53.3 10 33.3 2 6.7 2 6.7		
	Mean ± SD Min, Max		
Time post onset in days	1581 ± 1237 Min 421 Max 5087		

References

1. Hotton, M.; Huggons, E.; Hamlet, C.; Shore, D.; Johnson, D.; Norris, J.H.; Kilcoyne, S.; Dalton, L. The psychosocial impact of facial palsy: A systematic review. *Br. J. Health Psychol.* **2020**, *25*, 695–727. [CrossRef] [PubMed]
2. Heckmann, J.G.; Urban, P.P.; Pitz, S.; Guntinas-Lichius, O.; Gágyor, I. The Diagnosis and Treatment of Idiopathic Facial Paresis (Bell's Palsy). *Dtsch. Ärztebl.* **2019**, *116*, 692–702. [CrossRef] [PubMed]
3. Dobel, C.; Miltner, W.H.R.; Witte, O.W.; Volk, G.F.; Guntinas-Lichius, O. Emotionale Auswirkungen einer Fazialisparese. *Laryngo-Rhino-Otologie* **2013**, *92*, 9–23. [CrossRef] [PubMed]
4. Movérare, T.; Lohmander, A.; Hultcrantz, M.; Sjögreen, L. Peripheral facial palsy: Speech, communication and oral motor function. *Eur. Ann. Otorhinolaryngol. Head Neck Dis.* **2017**, *134*, 27–31. [CrossRef]
5. Dobel, C.; Guntinas-Lichius, O. Psychological Exploration of Emotional, Commuicative, and Social Impairments in Patients with Facial Impairments. In *Facial Nerve Disorders and Diseases*; Thieme: Stuttgart, Germany, 2016; pp. 184–191.
6. Coulson, S.E.; O'Dwyer, N.J.; Adams, R.D.; Croxson, G.R. Expression of Emotion and Quality of Life after Facial Nerve Paralysis. *Otol. Neurol.* **2004**, *25*, 1014–1019. [CrossRef]
7. Slattery, W.H.; Azizzadeh, B. Preface. In *The Facial Nerve*; Thieme: New York, NY, USA, 2014; p. IX.
8. Hamlet, C.; Williamson, H.; Hotton, M.; Rumsey, N. 'Your face freezes and so does your life': A qualitative exploration of adults' psychosocial experiences of living with acquired facial palsy. *Br. J. Health Psychol.* **2021**, *26*, 977–994. [CrossRef]
9. Ishii, L.E.; Godoy, A.; Encarnacion, C.O.; Byrne, P.J.; Boahene, K.D.; Ishii, M. Not Just Another Face in the Crowd: Society's Perceptions of Facial Paralysis. *Fac. Plast. Reconstr. Surg.* **2012**, *122*, 533–538. [CrossRef]
10. Ishii, L.E.; Godoy, A.; Encarnacion, C.O.; Byrne, P.J.; Boahene, K.D.O.; Ishii, M. What Faces Reveal: Impaired Affect Display in Facial Paralysis. *Laryngoscope* **2011**, *121*, 1138–1143. [CrossRef]

11. Parsa, K.M.; Hancock, M.; Nguy, P.L.; Donalek, H.M.; Wang, H.; Barth, J.; Reilly, M.J. Association of Facial Paralysis with Perceptions of Personality and Physical Traits. *JAMA Netw. Open* **2020**, *3*, e205495. [CrossRef]
12. Swift, P.; Bogart, K. A hidden community: Facial disfigurement as a globally neglected human rights issue. *J. Oral Biol. Craniofac. Res.* **2021**, *11*, 652–657. [CrossRef]
13. Volk, G.F.; Klingner, C.; Finkensieper, M.; Witte, O.W.; Guntinas-Lichius, O. Prognostication of recovery time after acute peripheral facial palsy: A prospective cohort study. *BMJ Open* **2013**, *3*, e003007. [CrossRef]
14. Moran, C.J.; Neely, J.G. Patterns of facial nerve synkinesis. *Laryngoscope* **1996**, *106*, 1491–1496. [CrossRef]
15. Husseman, J.; Mehta, R.P. Management of Synkinesis. *Fac. Plast. Surg.* **2008**, *24*, 242–249. [CrossRef]
16. Finkensieper, M.; Volk, G.F.; Guntinas-Lichius, O. Erkrankungen des Nervus facialis. *Laryngo-Rhino-Otologie* **2012**, *91*, 121–142. [CrossRef]
17. Santos, F.; Slattery, W.H. Physiology of the Facial Nerve. In *The Facial Nerve*; Thieme: New York, NY, USA, 2014; pp. 12–16.
18. Butler, D.P.; Morales, D.R.; Johnson, K.; Nduka, C. Facial palsy: When and why to refer for specialist care. *Brit. J. Gen. Pract.* **2019**, *69*, 579–580. [CrossRef]
19. Guntinas-Lichius, O.; Volk, G.F.; Olsen, K.D.; Mäkitie, A.A.; Silver, C.E.; Zafereo, M.E.; Rinaldo, A.; Randolph, G.W.; Simo, R.; Shaha, A.R.; et al. Faical nerve electrodiagnostics for patients with facial palsy: A clinical practice guideline. *Eur. Arch. Oto-Rhino-Laryngol.* **2020**, *277*, 1855–1874. [CrossRef]
20. De Jongh, F.W.; Sanches, E.E.; Luijmes, R.; Pouwels, S.; Ramnarain, D.; Beurskens, C.H.G.; Monstrey, S.J.; Marres, H.A.M.; Ingels, K.J.A.O. Cosmetic appreciation and emotional processing in patients with a peripheral facial palsy: A systematic review. *Neuropsychologia* **2021**, *158*, 107894. [CrossRef]
21. Kuttenreich, A.-M.; von Piekartz, H.; Heim, S. Emotionserkennung von Patienten bei Zustand nach Schlaganfall: Auswirkungen einer Gesichtslähmung—Eine Querschnittstudie. In *DGN-Kongress 2020–Abstracts*; Deutsche Gesellschaft für Neurologie e.V.: Berlin, Germany, 2020; pp. 179–180.
22. Kuttenreich, A.-M.; von Piekartz, H.; Heim, S. Is there a difference in Facial Emotion Recognition after Stroke with vs. without Central Facial Paresis? *Diagnostics*, 2022; under revision.
23. Kuttenreich, A.-M.; von Piekartz, H.; Volk, G.F.; Guntinas-Lichius, O.; Heim, S. Fazialisparesen und ihre Auswirkungen auf die Emotionserkennung. Deutsche Gesellschaft für Hals-Nasen-Ohren-Heilkunde, Kopf- und Halschirurgie e.V. *Laryngo-Rhino-Otologie* **2021**, *100*, S296–S297.
24. Yuvaraj, R.; Murugappan, M.; Norlinah, M.I.; Sundaraj, K.; Khairiyah, M. Review of Emotion Recognition in Stroke Patients. *Dement. Geriatr. Cogn. Disord.* **2013**, *36*, 179–196. [CrossRef]
25. Neal, D.T.; Chartrand, T.L. Embodied Emotion Perception: Amplifying and Dempening Facial Feedback Modulates Emotion Perception Accuracy. *Soc. Psychol. Personal. Sci.* **2011**, *2*, 673–678. [CrossRef]
26. Storbeck, F.; Schlegelmilch, K.; Streitberger, K.-J.; Sommer, W.; Ploner, C.J. Delayed recognition of emotional faical expressions in Bell's palsy. *Cortex* **2019**, *120*, 524–531. [CrossRef]
27. Konnerth, V.; Mohr, G.; von Piekartz, H. Fähigkeit von Patienten mit einer peripheren Fazialisparese zur Erkennung von Emotionen—Eine Pilotstudie. *Rehabilitation* **2016**, *55*, 19–25. [CrossRef]
28. Korb, S.; Wood, A.; Banks, C.A.; Agoulnik, D.; Hadlock, T.A.; Niedenthal, P.M. Asymmetry of Facial Mimicry and Emotion Perception in Patients with Unilateral Facial Paralysis. *JAMA Fac. Plast. Surg.* **2016**, *18*, 222–227. [CrossRef]
29. Kret, M.E.; de Gelder, B. A review on sex differences in processing emotional signals. *Neuropsychologia* **2012**, *50*, 1211–1221. [CrossRef]
30. Wingenbach, T.S.H.; Ashwin, C.; Brosnan, M. Sex differences in facial emotion recognition across varying expression intensity leves from videos. *PLoS ONE* **2018**, *13*, e0190634. [CrossRef]
31. Ruffman, T.; Henry, J.D.; Livingstone, V.; Phillips, L.H. A meta-analytic review of emotion recognition and aging: Implications for neuropsychological models of aging. *Neurosci. Behav. Rev.* **2008**, *4*, 863–881. [CrossRef] [PubMed]
32. Kessels, R.P.C.; Montagne, B.; Hendriks, A.W.; Perrett, D.I.; de Haan, E.H.F. Assessment of perception of morphed facial expressions using the Emotion Recognition Task: Normative data from healthy participants aged 8–75. *J. Neuropsychol.* **2014**, *8*, 75–93. [CrossRef] [PubMed]
33. Ross, B.G.; Fradet, G.; Nedzelski, J.M. Development of a sensitive clinical facial grading system. *Otolaryngol. Head Neck Surg.* **1996**, *114*, 380–386. [CrossRef]
34. Neumann, T.; Lorenz, A.; Volk, G.F.; Hamzei, F.; Schulz, S.; Guntinas-Lichius, O. Validierung einer Deutschen Version des Sunnybrook Facial Grading Systems. *Laryngo-Rhino-Otologie* **2017**, *96*, 168–174. [CrossRef] [PubMed]
35. House, J.W.; Brackmann, D.E. Facial nerve grading system. *Otolaryngol.-Head Neck Surg.* **1985**, *93*, 146–147. [CrossRef] [PubMed]
36. Ekman, P. Universal Facial Expressions of Emotion. *Calif. Mental Health Res. Dig.* **1970**, *8*, 151–158.
37. Ekman, P. An argument for basic emotions. *Cogn. Emot.* **1992**, *6*, 169–200. [CrossRef]
38. Levenson, R.W. Basic Emotion Questions. *Emot. Rev.* **2011**, *3*, 379–386. [CrossRef]
39. Babbage, D.R.; Yim, J.; Zupan, B.; Neumann, D.; Tomita, M.R.; Willer, B. Meta-Analysis of Facial Affect Recognition Difficulties after Traumatic Brain Injury. *Neuropsychology* **2011**, *25*, 277–285. [CrossRef]
40. Myfacetraining. Available online: https://www.myfacetraining.com/ (accessed on 9 April 2022).
41. CRAFTA Cranio Facial Therapy Academy. Operating Guidelines CRAFTA Facemirroring Assessment and Treatment. Available online: https://www.myfacetraining.com/downloads/CRAFTA%20Operating%20Guidelines.pdf (accessed on 25 March 2022).

42. Belin, P.; Fillion-Bilodeau, S.; Gosselin, F. The Montreal Affective Voices: A validated set of nonverbal affect bursts for research on auditory affecitve processing. *Behav. Res. Methods* **2008**, *40*, 531–539. [CrossRef]
43. Peirce, J.; MacAskill, M. *Building Experiments in PsychoPy*; Sage: London, UK, 2018.
44. Microsoft Corporation. Microsoft Excel 2019. Available online: https://office.microsoft.com/excel (accessed on 1 January 2019).
45. International Business Machines Corporation. *IBM Statistics for Windows, Version 28.0*; IBM Corp.: North Castle, NY, USA, 2021.
46. Vrabec, J.T.; Backous, D.D.; Djalilian, H.R.; Gidley, P.W.; Leonetti, J.P.; Marzo, S.J.; Morrison, D.; Ng, M.; Ramsey, M.J.; Schaitkin, B.M.; et al. Facial Nerve Grading System 2.0. *Otolaryngol.-Head Neck Surg.* **2009**, *140*, 445–450.
47. Coles, N.A.; Larsen, J.T.; Lench, H.C. A Meta-Analysis of the Facial Feedback Literature: Effects of Facial Feedback on Emotion Experience Are Small and Variable. *Psychol. Bull.* **2019**, *145*, 610–651. [CrossRef]
48. Hawk, S.T.; Fischer, A.H.; van Kleef, G.A. Face the Noise: Embodied Response to Nonverbal Vocalizations of Discrete Emotions. *J. Personal. Soc. Psychol.* **2012**, *102*, 796–814. [CrossRef]
49. Baumeister, J.-C.; Papa, G.; Foroni, F. Deeper than skin deep—The effect of botulinum toxin-A on emotion processing. *Toxicon* **2016**, *118*, 86–90. [CrossRef]
50. Schirmer, A. Is the voice an auditory face? An ALE meta-analysis comparing vocal and facial emotion processing. *Soc. Cogn. Affect. Neurosci.* **2018**, *13*, 1–13. [CrossRef]
51. Adolphs, R. Neural systems for recognizing emotion. *Curr. Opin. Neurobiol.* **2002**, *12*, 169–177. [CrossRef]
52. Kuhn, L.K.; Wydell, T.; Lavan, N.; McGettigan, C.; Garrido, L. Similar Representations of Emotions across Faces and Voices. *Emotion* **2017**, *17*, 912–937. [CrossRef]
53. Weisgerber, A.; Vermeulen, N.; Peretz, I.; Samson, S.; Philippot, P.; Marauge, P.; D'Aoust, C.d.; de Jaegere, A.; Delatte, B.; Gillain, B.; et al. Facial, vocal and musical emotion recognition is altered in paranoid schizophrenic patients. *Psychiatry Res.* **2015**, *229*, 188–193. [CrossRef]
54. Schirmer, A.; Adolphs, R. Emotion Perception from Face, Voice, and Touch: Comparisions and Convergence. *Trends Cogn. Sci.* **2017**, *21*, 216–228. [CrossRef]
55. Du, S.; Tao, Y.; Martinez, A.M. Compound facial expressions of emotion. *Proc. Natl. Acad. Sci. USA* **2014**, *111*, e1454–e1462. [CrossRef]
56. Sato, W.; Krumhuber, E.G.; Jellema, T.; Williams, J.H.G. *Dynamic Emotional Communication*; Frontiers Media SA: Lausanne, Switzerland, 2020.
57. Ruba, A.L.; Pollak, S.D. Children's emotion inferences from masked faces: Implications for social interactions during COVID-19. *PLoS ONE* **2020**, *15*, e0243708. [CrossRef]
58. Gori, M.; Schiatti, L.; Amadeo, M.B. Masking Emotions: Face Masks Impair How We Read Emotions. *Front. Psychol.* **2021**, *12*, 1541. [CrossRef]
59. Wan, J.; Lai, Z.; Liu, J.; Zhou, J.; Gao, C. Robust Face Alignment by Multi-Order High-Precision Hourglass Network. *IEEE Trans. Image Process.* **2020**, *30*, 121–133. [CrossRef] [PubMed]
60. Guarin, D.L.; Yunusova, Y.; Taati, B.; Dusselderp, J.R.; Mohan, S.; Tavares, J.; van Veen, M.M.; Fortier, E.; Hadlock, T.A.; Jowett, N. Toward an Automatic System for Computer-Aided Assessment in Facial Palsy. *Fac. Plast. Surg. Aesthet. Med.* **2020**, *22*, 42–49. [CrossRef] [PubMed]
61. Miller, M.Q.; Hadlock, T.A.; Fortier, E.; Guarin, D.L. The Auto-eFACE: Machine Learning-Enhanced Program Yields Automated Facial Palsy Assessment Tool. *Plast. Reconstr. Surg.* **2021**, *147*, 467–474. [CrossRef] [PubMed]
62. Parra-Dominguez, G.S.; Sanchez-Yanez, R.E.; Garcia-Capulin, C.H. Facial Paralysis Detection on Images Using Key Point Analysis. *Appl. Sci.* **2021**, *11*, 2435. [CrossRef]
63. Volk, G.F.; Thielker, J.; Mothes, O.; Guntinas-Lichius, O. Objective Measurment of Outcomes in Facial Palsy. In *Management of Post-Facial Paralysis Synkinesis*; Elsevier: Amsterdam, The Netherlands, 2021; pp. 59–74.
64. Mothes, O.; Modersohn, L.; Volk, G.F.; Klingner, C.; Witte, O.W.; Schlattmann, P.; Denzler, J.; Guntinas-Lichius, O. Automated objective and marker-free facial grading using photographs of patients with facial palsy. *Eur. Arch. Oto-Rhino-Laryngol.* **2019**, *276*, 3335–3343. [CrossRef]
65. Thielker, J.; Kuttenreich, A.-M.; Volk, G.F.; Guntinas-Lichius, O. Idiopathische Fazialisparese (Bell-Parese): Aktueller Stand in Diagnostik und Therapie. *Laryngo-Rhino-Otologie* **2021**, *100*, 1004–1018. [CrossRef]

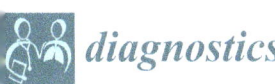

Case Report

Reanimation of the Smile with Neuro-Vascular Anastomosed Gracilis Muscle: A Case Series

Helen Abing *,†, Carina Pick †, Tabea Steffens, Jenny Shachi Sharma, Jens Peter Klußmann and Maria Grosheva *

Department of Otorhinolaryngology, Head and Neck Surgery, Faculty of Medicine, University of Cologne, 50937 Cologne, Germany; carina.pick@gmx.de.de (C.P.); tabea.steffens@t-online.de (T.S.); shachi.sharma@uk-koeln.de (J.S.S.); jens.klußmann@uk-koeln.de (J.P.K.)
* Correspondence: helen.abing@uk-koeln.de (H.A.); maria.grosheva@uk-koeln.de (M.G.)
† These authors contributed equally to this work.

Abstract: Background: The aim of our manuscript was to evaluate the time course of clinical and electromyographical (EMG) reinnervation after the reanimation of the smile using a gracilis muscle transplant which is reinnervated with the masseteric nerve. Methods: We present a case series of five patients with a longstanding peripheral facial palsy, who underwent a reanimation of the lower face using a gracilis muscle transplant with masseteric nerve reinnervation from June 2019 to October 2020. Trial-specific follow-up examinations were carried out every three months using clinical assessment and EMG, up to 12 months after the surgery. The grading was carried out using the House–Brackmann scale (HB), the Stennert Index, and a self-designed Likert-like scale for graft reinnervation and smile excursion. Results: The surgery was feasible in all of the patients. The reanimation was performed under general anesthesia in an inpatient setting. Postoperative complications which resulted in prolonged hospitalization occurred in two of the five patients. All of the patients showed a preoperative flaccid facial palsy. The first single reinnervation potentials were detected 3.1 ± 0.1 months after surgery. After 5.6 (±1.4) months, in three (3/5) patients, clear reinnervation patterns were present. Clinically, the patients obtained symmetry of the face at rest after 5.6 (±1.4) months, and could spontaneously smile without the co-activation of the jaw after an average time of 10.8 (±1.8) months. All of the patients were able to express a spontaneous emotion-stimulated smile after one year. Conclusion: Micro-neurovascular gracilis muscle transfer reinnervated with a masseteric nerve is a sufficient and reliable rehabilitation technique for the lower face, and is performed as a single-stage surgery. The nerve supply via the masseteric nerve allows the very rapid and strong reinnervation of the graft, and results in a spontaneous smile within 10 months.

Keywords: longstanding facial palsy; gracilis transfer; masseteric nerve; needle electromyography; outcome

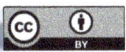

1. Introduction

Peripheral facial nerve palsy is the most common peripheral cranial nerve disorder. Its etiology is very diverse. Although the most common, idiopathic facial nerve palsy (FP) (Bell's palsy, with 60–75% of all cases) heals in nearly 80–90% of patients, other etiologies are known to be associated with defective healing, or even to result in a longstanding flaccid paralysis [1]. FP dramatically limits the quality of life on various levels. Dysphagia, speech disorders, xerophthalmia and consecutive corneal damage are some but not all of the possible physical consequences of the FP. Furthermore, limited nonverbal communication and the change of the appearance of the face significantly impact daily life. As a consequence, patients often suffer from psychological stress and social isolation [2]. For both aspects, the proper function of the lower face, especially the existence of the spontaneous smile, is crucial [3].

Surgical nerve reconstruction and reconstructive surgery are considered to be the gold standard for the reanimation of longstanding FP [3]. However, as structurally irreversible changes occur in the facial musculature, facial nerve fibers and the synaptic connections within the first 2–3 years after the palsy's onset, the reanimation of a longstanding paralysis requires complex surgical procedures [4]. For the reanimation of the smile, the transfer of the gracilis muscle, which then mimics the function of the zygomatic muscle, is internationally established. Previous studies have demonstrated the benefit of this procedure due to improvement of functional aspects, a positive effect on social interaction and self-acceptance, and an increase in quality of life [5]. Muscle transfer using a gracilis graft was first described by Harii et al. in 1976 [6]. Here, nerval reinnervation via cross-face transfer was considered the most advantageous [6]. The procedure is associated with good motor function, the almost symmetrical mobility of the face, and simultaneous control via the facial nerve of the opposite side [7,8]. However, this reanimation technique requires multi-stage surgery, and is associated with the partial sacrifice of the healthy facial nerve branches, which might result in synkinesis.

The reinnervation of the gracilis graft with the masseteric nerve represents an alternative approach. The harvesting of the muscle graft and the reinnervation can be achieved during a single stage operation. The nerve is accessible in the already exposed surgical site [9,10]. Motor unit reinnervation is expected to be faster due to the shorter innervation distance compared to the facial nerve [11]. However, for a good functional outcome, the contraction of the gracilis graft has to be triggered by biting, which requires the sufficient compliance of the patient during rehabilitation as well as the sufficient plasticity of the brain [12–14]. In more than half of the cases, a spontaneous, emotionally stimulated smile can be obtained without the use of biting or chewing [15].

The aim of our manuscript was to describe the surgical procedure and the time-course of clinical and electromyographical reinnervation after the reanimation of the smile using a gracilis muscle transplant, which was reinnervated with the masseteric nerve.

2. Patients and Methods

We present a case series of 5 patients with a longstanding peripheral facial palsy, who underwent a reanimation of the lower face using a gracilis muscle transplant with masseteric nerve reinnervation from June 2019 to October 2020. We analyzed the time course of the reinnervation of the gracilis muscle and the final functional outcome after one year.

All of the patients signed a written consent form for data collection. Only adult patients with a longstanding facial nerve palsy were included. The study was approved by the Ethics Committee of the University of Cologne (approval Nr. 22-1106-retro, Cologne, Germany).

2.1. Surgery

All of the patients underwent the surgical procedure under general anesthesia in an inpatient setting. All of the operations were carried out by surgeons MG and SJS in a simultaneous two-team approach.

First, the dissection of the face and the parotid area was carried out (MG). The vessels including the retromandibular vein plexus and superficial temporal artery were identified after the preauricular incision. Then, the masseteric triangle—including the zygomatic bone, the buccal branch of the facial nerve, and the mandibular joint—was exposed [16,17]. The masseteric nerve was identified and dissected to the maximum extent. For the positioning of the gracilis graft, the subcutaneous tissue of the cheek was mobilized to the nasolabial fold, and further to the oral commissure. The dissection was carried out in a sub-SMAS deep plain. During the subcutaneous dissection of the lower and upper lip, the orbicularis oris muscle (OOM) was identified. In order to enable the tissue dissection and future positioning of the gracilis muscle, skin incisions along the nasolabial fold and submentally were carried out.

The second surgical team (SJS) harvested the gracilis muscle together with the neurovascular pedicle, including the obturator nerve and a branch of the medial circumflex femoral artery or of the profunda femoris artery. The muscle was removed in its entire width.

For the positioning of the graft, the inferior part of the muscle was separated into two equal pedicles. The superior part of the muscle included the recipient vessels and the obturator nerve (Figure 1). First, the microsurgical end-to-end suture of the masseteric and obturator nerve was carried out using non-resorbable Ethilon 9-0 (Ethicon®, Johnson & Johnson Medical GmbH, Norderstedt, Germany) sutures. The donor artery (the superficial temporal artery) was sutured end-to-end to the recipient artery using Ethilon 9-0 sutures. For the venous anastomosis (retromandibular vein), a coupler system (Gem Coupler®, Baxter Healthcare, Opfikon, Switzerland) was used (Figure 2). In one patient, we chose the facial artery and vein as donor vessels. The muscle graft was positioned in such way that the peripheral pedicles reached the OOM medially. The muscle pedicles were sutured to the OOM fibers of the upper and lower lip with non-resorbable sutures (Ethibond 4-0, Ethicon®). The united pedicles were also sutured to the OOM in the oral commissure. We used a micro-osteosynthesis 5- to 4-hole plate (KLS Martin Group) to attach the superior part of the muscle graft to the zygomatic bone. A wound drain was placed in both surgical areas. Wound closure was performed in layers using subcutaneous and skin sutures.

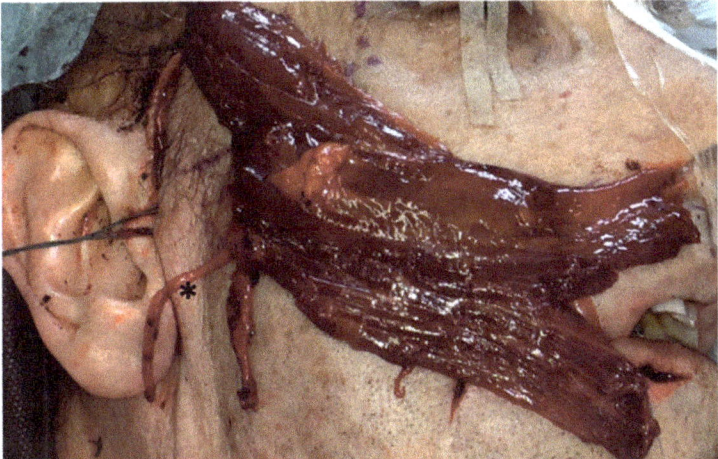

Figure 1. The gracilis muscle graft before implantation in the planned orientation on the right side. * marks the obturator nerve.

In some patients, additional static reanimation procedures of the upper face were carried out during the same operation. These were forehead and brow lifts, eyelid loading, and lateral canthopexy.

2.2. Data Assessment and Follow-Up

Data on the patients' characteristics, the surgery duration in minutes, the duration of the hospitalization, and data on postoperative complications were assessed.

Trial-specific follow-up examinations were carried out every three to four months. Facial function was documented preoperatively and during the follow-up visits. The grading was carried out using the House–Brackmann scale (HB) and the Stennert Index [18]. The Stennert Index allows the grading of the resting face (0 for regular function to 4 for flaccid complete paralysis) and during voluntary movement (0 for no paresis and 6 for complete flaccid paralysis) [18]. As neither scale (the Stennert Index nor the HB Scale) was originally designed to evaluate facial symmetry after reconstruction, we used the Likert-like scale to evaluate the clinical outcome. Clinical outcomes were documented as follows: asymmetry at rest, flaccid paralysis; asymmetry at rest, minimal improvement of the muscle tone while biting; improved muscle tone and symmetry at rest while biting; symmetry at rest while biting, spontaneous smile possible; symmetry at rest, spontaneous smile without biting.

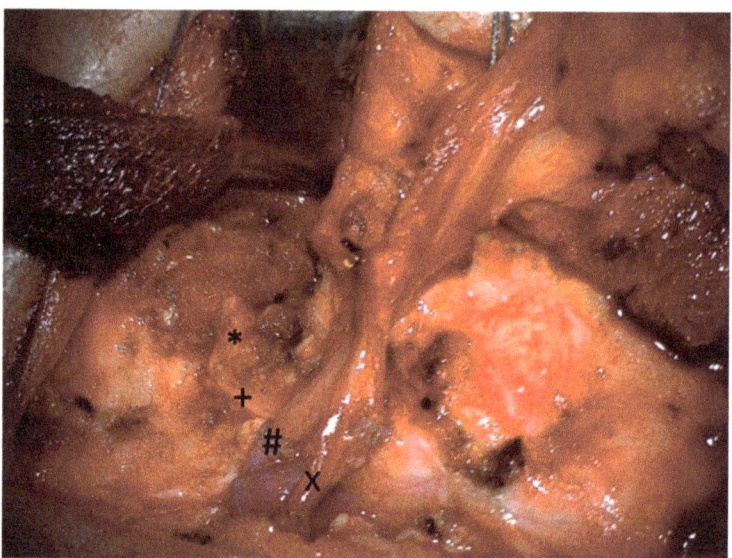

Figure 2. Operative situs on the right side after the completion of the nerve and vessel sutures using the superficial temporal artery and retromandibular vein. * marks the masseteric nerve, + marks the obturator nerve, # marks venous anastomosis, and x marks the arterial anastomosis.

Needle electromyography (EMG) was carried out during each follow-up examination until the primary outcome (the clear excursion of the smile) was clearly visible (Nicolet Electromygoraphy®, Natus Medical, San Carlos, CA, USA). The EMG results were rated as follows: preoperative EMG, no activity; single reinnervation potentials while biting; single reinnervation potentials during smiling without biting; clear reinnervation pattern without biting; clear clinical reinnervation, no EMG examination necessary.

2.3. Statistical Analysis

The statistical analysis was performed using SPSS software, version 28.0 (IBM Corporation, Armonk, New York, NY, USA). We present the quantitative variables as the mean ± SD, and the qualitative variables as absolute numbers and percent values.

3. Results

3.1. Characteristics of the Patients and Surgery

From June 2019 to October 2020, five patients underwent the reanimation procedure. The characteristics of the patients are shown in Table 1. The patients, three of them female, were 48.7 ± 16.1 years old. The median duration of paralysis was 18.9 years (range 2–55 years). The paralysis was on the right side of the face in all of the patients. Three patients showed complete flaccid paralysis before the surgery. One patient showed a paralysis score of HB IV, for a good resting tone of the facial muscles. Another patient consulted us because of congenital middle face dysplasia and showed a facial palsy with an HB score of V, with preserved function of the frontalis muscle. Preoperative needle EMG showed no voluntary activity of the nasalis and zygomatic muscles, nor of the depressor anguli oris muscle (DAOM) in any of the patients.

Table 1. Patients' characteristics.

Patient	Gender	Age in Years	Duration of Palsy in Years	Etiology	Preoperative Facial Grading (House Brackmann (HB) Score)
1	male	68.1	2.0	Radical parotidectomy and postoperative Radiation, Parotid Carcinoma	VI
2	female	48.6	10.5	Idiopatic	VI
3	male	48.0	23.1	Vestibular Schwannoma	VI
4	female	23.8	4.1	Facial Nerve Schwannoma	IV
5	female	55.0	55.1	Congenital dysplasia of the middle and lower face	V

The surgical procedure, as described above, was feasible in all of the patients. The mean duration of the surgery was 506 (±62.5) minutes, and the mean duration of the hospitalization was 11 (±3.7) days. Two patients were hospitalized longer because of a postoperative complication (patient 1: massive hemorrhage into the thigh because of derailed anticoagulation; patient 3: delayed wound healing). Patient 5 had prolonged postoperative ventilation due to a complex dysplasia of the middle and lower face.

For vascular anastomosis, we chose the superficial temporal artery and retromandibular vein as donor vessels in four cases because of the good accessibility in the already-opened surgical site. In patient 1, these vessels were not preserved during previous surgery for parotid cancer. For this reason, we chose the facial artery and vein as donors.

3.2. Follow-Up and Outcome

The follow-up took place every 3.1 (±1.1) months, on average. The first follow-up took place after 3.1 (±1.0) months, and the last follow-up took place after 12.3 (±3.0) months. The timeline of the visits is displayed in Table 2.

Table 2. Follow-up timeline in months, average.

Follow-Up Visit	Time from Surgery, Months (±SD)	Time to Previous Visit, Months (±SD)
1	3.1 (1.0)	3.2 (±1.0)
2	5.6 (1.4)	2.5 (±0.6)
3	8.4 (2.0)	2.8 (±0.9)
4	10.8 (1.8)	3.1 (±0.7)
5	16.1 (0.4)	4.9 (±2.5)

The functional outcomes and EMG results are summarized in Figures 3 and 4, respectively. The first improvement of the musculature's tone was detected at the first follow-up, after an average time of 3.1 (±1.0) months. At this stage, asymmetry at rest was still evident, and the masseter muscle was needed to increase the muscle tone by biting. Symmetry at rest was present on average at the time of the second follow-up visit after 5.6 (±1.4) months. All of the patients showed symmetry at rest and a spontaneous smile without the use of the jaw at the time of the fourth follow-up (average 10.8 (±1.8) months).

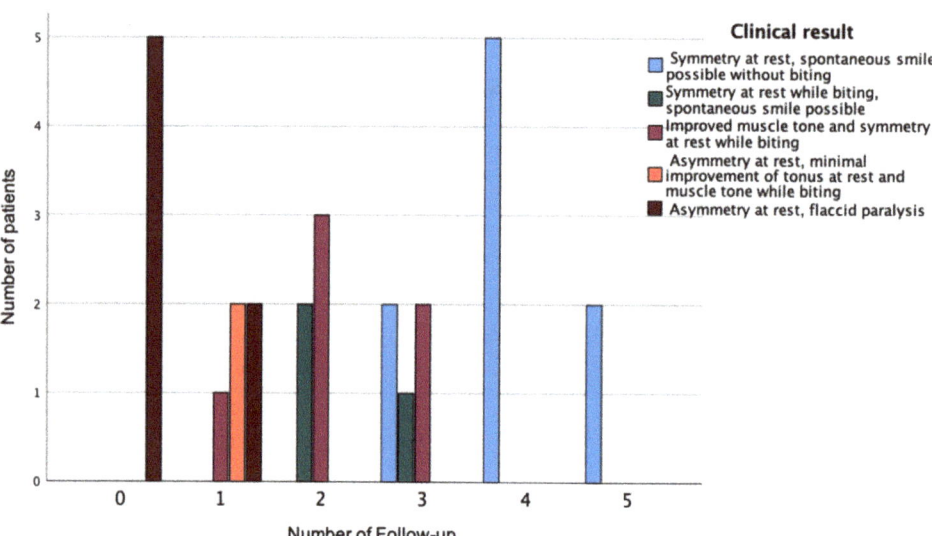

Figure 3. Functional outcome at the first to fifth follow-up visit. 0 = preoperative state, 1–5 = number of the follow-up visit.

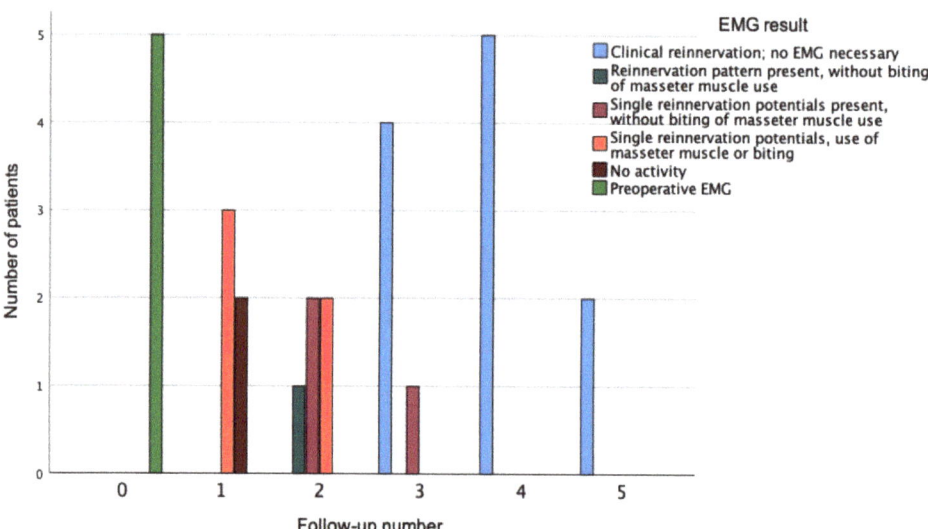

Figure 4. EMG-result at the first to fifth follow-up visit. 0 = preoperative state, 1–5 = number of the follow-up visit.

Needle-EMG examinations were carried out during each examination until a spontaneous smile was obvious. The first reinnervation potentials were detected earliest at the first follow-up visit in three patients (Figure 4). At the second follow-up, after 5.6 (±1.4) months, three patients showed reinnervation patterns without the use of the jaw or biting. At the time of the third follow-up (8.4 (±2.0) months), a spontaneous smile was possible and no EMG was needed.

3.3. Clinical Outcome

All of the patients demonstrated a spontaneous smile by one year after surgery. Table 3 and Figures 5 and 6 demonstrate the clinical outcome of the patients before surgery and at the one-year follow-up appointment. Both global palsy scores improved significantly after the surgery. However, several additional static procedures were carried out in each of the patients (Table 3).

Table 3. Facial paralysis scores, preoperatively and at the last (one-year) follow-up appointment.

Patient	Timepoint of Documentation	House Brackmann Score	Stennert Index	Additional Surgical Procedures
1	Preoperative	6	4/6	Forehead-/Browlift, Lidloading
	Last follow-up	2	0/3	
2	Preoperative	6	4/6	Forehead-/Browlift
	Last follow-up	2	1/1	
3	Preoperative	6	4/6	Canthopexy, Lidloading
	Last follow-up	3	1/4	
4	Preoperative	4	3/5	Canthopexy, Lidloading
	Last follow-up	2	1/1	
5	Preoperative	5	3/4	-
	Last follow-up	3	2/1	

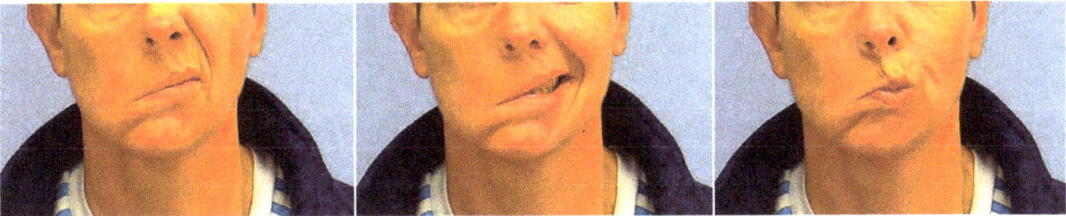

Figure 5. Preoperative excursion of the mouth in patient 4. **Left**: wrinkling the nose; **center**: smiling; **right**: pointing the mouth.

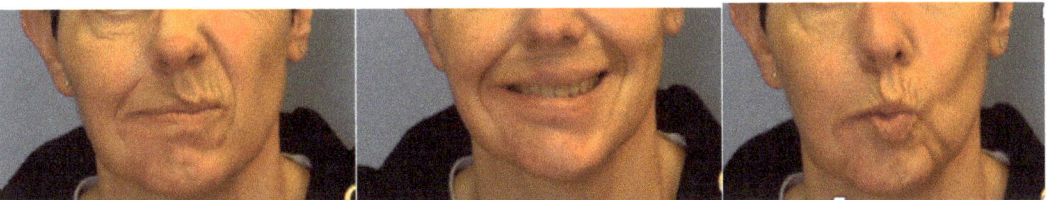

Figure 6. Postoperative result 16 months after the procedure in patient 4. **Left**: wrinkling the nose; **center**: smiling; **right**: pointing the mouth.

4. Discussion

In the present study, we investigated the time course of reinnervation and the functional outcome after the reanimation of the lower face with a micro-neurovascular anastomosed gracilis muscle flap, supplied by the masseteric nerve. Five patients with longstanding FP, who underwent the surgery between June 2019 and October 2020, were consecutively followed up over the time period of one year. The time course of the gracilis graft reinnervation was observed clinically, and was examined using a needle EMG.

The major decision points for the reanimation technique were: 1/ one-stage surgery; 2/ the unclear condition of the peripheral facial nerve branches after previous tumor surgery (Patient 1); and 3/ the fiber quality of the masseteric nerve (stronger or wider excursion of the smile). Besides patient 1, all of the patients preferred a single-stage surgery and did not wish to undergo a cross-face reanimation of the gracilis graft. In addition, some patients seemed to prefer the sacrifice of the masseteric function over the facial nerve branches of the healthy side, as is the case with cross-face treatment.

All of the patients showed a preoperative flaccid facial palsy. All of them were able to express a spontaneous emotion-stimulated smile after one year. We noticed a very short reinnervation interval in our patients. The first single reinnervation potentials were detected 3 months after surgery. After 6 months, in three (3/5) patients, clear reinnervation patterns were present in the gracilis graft, which did not require the co-activation of the masseteric muscles (using chewing or biting). Clinically, the patients obtained symmetry of the face at rest after 6 months, and could spontaneously smile without the co-activation of the jaw after an average time of 11 months. In the context of grading, the clinical appearance corresponded to an improvement of two to four points in both the HB and Stennert index. The postoperative outcome was significantly improved in 100% of the cases. This corresponds to the empirical values of other studies [19,20]. Compared to the cross-face reinnervated gracilis graft, in which a good functional outcome can be expected after a period of up to 18 months [8], the patients with a masseteric nerve-supplied gracilis graft achieved the final result considerably earlier. Although all of the patients could express a spontaneous smile in our case series, the co-activation of the jaw and the masseteric muscles is essential to support reinnervation. For this reason, the rehabilitation might be challenging for patients with a lower motivation for training, with a weak muscle tonus, or who are not able to chew or bite (i.e., non-functional dental status). The cross-face transfer, on the other hand, enables the simultaneous control of the muscles due to simultaneous nerve supply, and enables symmetrical mobility [8,19]. Therefore, cross-face supplied gracilis transfer is still considered to be the gold standard for the reanimation of the lower face, especially in young patients [17,21]. Our patients underwent a postoperative physical therapy program to stimulate reinnervation and to increase muscle tonus as soon as the reinnervation pattern was detectable in the EMG. We recommend the use of EMG diagnostics for the early detection of the reinnervation potentials, so that physical therapy is initiated as early as possible. However, some patients might profit from the additional stimulation training of the graft, i.e., electrical stimulation to obtain higher muscle tone and volume [22,23].

Previously published data are inconsistent and ambiguous regarding the ability to develop a spontaneous, emotionally stimulated smile after reconstruction with a free muscle graft innervated via the masseteric nerve. Some studies describe the nerval reinnervation via cross-face transfer as the only option for emotionally stimulated mobility. Bigliolo et al. reported a spontaneous smile after reconstruction via the masseteric nerve in about 10% of the patients [24]. However, there are number of studies which report far better results. For example, Hontanilla et al. described the achievement of spontaneous mobility in 55% of their patients [15], and Manktelow et al. reported success in 60% of their cases [11].

Our case series included a somewhat-young patient collective. The good plasticity of the brain might explain the success of the procedure. Another possible explanation for the good outcome might be the close and even overlapping cortical relationship of the responsible cortical areas for smiling and biting. In particular, women and young patients were described to obtain a favorable outcome and good functional results [15].

Compared to the cross-face transfer of the gracilis graft, the masseteric nerve transfer still poses a one-stage surgery and is best suited for patients who wish to obtain a quicker result and a single-surgery procedure. As the gracilis graft only simulates the direction of the zygomatic muscle, we observed a postoperative hollowness of the periorbital region. The patients have to be informed about the possible further treatments of procedures, which might be necessary in the further course of therapy (augmentation, etc.). Furthermore, the paresis of the upper face was not treated here. Therefore, the rehabilitation of the eye region (i.e., lidloading, eyebrow lift, etc.) is often additionally necessary. As mentioned on page 3, four patients underwent supplementary static procedures such as brow lifts, lidloading or lateral canthopexy. The additional procedures for each patient are also named in Table 3, on page 9. These procedures were crucial for the improvement of the ocular closure and overall facial symmetry.

The dynamic rehabilitation of the eye region is also possible. We prefer the dynamic reanimation of the eye closure (mostly the transposition of the temporal muscle) as a second step of facial reanimation if static procedures do not lead to satisfactory results. Especially in younger patients, static lidloading or brow lifts are easy and quick techniques with good, long-lasting results. In older patients, we would probably recommend dynamic eye rehabilitation, which is slightly more time-consuming, but generally leads to a better long-term result.

Besides the gracilis graft, the common alternatives for muscle replacement are the minor pectoralis, anterior serratus and latissimus dorsi muscles [25].

The gracilis muscle, however, has become the most common muscle graft because of its accessibility, superficial course, and the low morbidity of the sampling site [7,8,11,17,20]. The simultaneous surgical approach of both sites, the face and the thigh, is possible in a two-team approach.

In our case series, we mostly used the superficial temporal artery and the retromandibular vein plexus as donor vessels for the muscle graft. Despite the small vessel calibers, the blood supply was sufficient in all of the cases. In comparative studies, the facial artery and vein are preferred because of their larger caliber. In 20%, the facial vessels are dissected in the submental triangle. We also used the facial vessel supply in one patient after a radical parotid surgery because the superficial temporal artery was not present. However, in approximately 33% of the patients with preexisting (tumor) surgery, even the facial artery and vein are no longer available, such that alternative blood donors have to be considered [26]. In this case, the submental vessels might be a good donor replacement [27]. Furthermore, it is important to acknowledge that the changed anatomy after radical resection might pose a challenge in the visualization of the anatomical structures. In the case of our patient with a congenital dysplasia of the middle face, the dissection of the masseteric nerve was more difficult but still feasible.

Faris et al. also described this procedure to be advantageous in patients with FP after radical parotid surgery [9]. Besides the beneficial access to the donor nerve and rapid reinnervation of the graft, the muscle bulk also acts as a kind of filling material after a radical resection of tissue, and improves the symmetry of the face. Furthermore, the fiber quality of the masseteric nerve leads to more powerful reinnervation compared to the cross-face transfer [8].

Postoperative complications occurred in two of our five cases. One patient developed a wound infection of the cheek, which led to a prolonged hospitalization. Another patient underwent a revision surgery of the thigh and neck because of postoperative bleeding which occurred due to an overdose of anticoagulation therapy during his ICU stay. The literature search revealed only few studies which systematically report on complications. Garcia et al. described, in their meta-analysis, an overall complication rate of 9.6%. The majority of the complications were mild, such as wound infections in 3.5 to 5.6%, and hematomas in 3.6% of the cases. Flap failure occurred in 1.8% of cases [20,28].

In summary, dynamic facial reanimation with a free gracilis transfer is a valuable technique to improve oral competence and emotional and nonverbal communication. An improvement in facial symmetry, as well as an increase in quality of life, occured in 100% of the cases with successful muscle transfer, regardless of the choice of donor nerve [19,20]. Hontanilla et al. even discussed whether the treatment with the masseteric nerve should be the preferred alternative when considering all of the advantages, such as the lower donor site morbidity, a more symmetrical and stronger smile, and—in the course of time—also a possible spontaneous mobility [8]. In summary, we consider the micro-neurovascular anastomosed grafting with the gracilis muscle and masseteric nerve to be a sufficient and reliable rehabilitation option for the lower face. Furthermore, considering the increasing data on this topic, we believe that a spontaneous smile is a realistic goal in facial paralysis reanimation with the masseteric nerve. A drawback of our study is the limited number of cases. Therefore, larger numbers of patients are required in order to draw general conclusions.

5. Conclusions

In conclusion, micro-neurovascular anastomosed grafting using the gracilis muscle flap is a sufficient and reliable rehabilitation option for the lower face. The nerve supply via the masseteric nerve allows the very rapid and strong reinnervation of the face, and results in a spontaneous smile within 10 months of the surgery.

Author Contributions: Conceptualization, H.A. and M.G..; methodology, M.G.; software, T.S., H.A. and M.G.; validation, H.A., C.P. and M.G.; formal analysis, T.S. and H.A.; investigation, H.A., C.P. and M.G.; resources, M.G. and J.P.K.; data curation, T.S. and H.A.; writing—original draft preparation, H.A. and C.P.; writing—review and editing, J.S.S., J.P.K. and M.G.; visualization, M.G.; supervision, J.S.S. and M.G.; project administration, J.S.S., J.P.K. and M.G.; All authors have read and agreed to the published version of the manuscript.

Funding: This research received no external funding.

Institutional Review Board Statement: The study was conducted in accordance with the Declaration of Helsinki, and approved by the Institutional Ethics Committee of the University of Cologne (approval Nr. 22-1106-retro, Cologne, Germany).

Informed Consent Statement: Informed consent was obtained from all subjects involved in the study.

Conflicts of Interest: The authors declare no conflict of interest. The funders had no role in the design of the study; in the collection, analyses, or interpretation of data; in the writing of the manuscript, or in the decision to publish the results.

References

1. Heckmann, J.G.; Urban, P.P.; Pitz, S.; Guntinas-Lichius, O.; Gágyor, I. The Diagnosis and Treatment of Idiopathic Facial Paresis (Bell's Palsy). *Dtsch. Arztebl. Int.* **2019**, *116*, 692–702. [CrossRef] [PubMed]
2. Slattery, W.H.; Azizzadeh, B. *The Facial Nerve*; Thieme: New York, NY, USA, 2014.
3. May, M.; Schaitkin, B.M. *Facial Paralysis: Rehabilitation Techniques*; Thieme: New York, NY, USA, 2003.
4. Guntinas-Lichius, O.; Streppel, M.; Stennert, E. Postoperative functional evaluation of different reanimation techniques for facial nerve repair. *Am. J. Surg.* **2006**, *191*, 61–67. [CrossRef] [PubMed]
5. Guntinas-Lichius, O. Reconstructive surgery for patients with facial palsy. *Laryngorhinootologie* **2009**, *88*, 544–551. [CrossRef] [PubMed]
6. Harii, K. Microneurovascular free muscle transplantation for reanimation of facial paralysis. *Clin. Plast. Surg.* **1979**, *6*, 361–375. [CrossRef]
7. Gasteratos, K.; Azzawi, S.A.; Vlachopoulos, N.; Lese, I.; Spyropoulou, G.A.; Grobbelaar, A.O. Workhorse Free Functional Muscle Transfer Techniques for Smile Reanimation in Children with Congenital Facial Palsy: Case Report and Systematic Review of the Literature. *J. Plast. Reconstr. Aesthet. Surg.* **2021**, *74*, 1423–1435. [CrossRef] [PubMed]
8. Hontanilla, B.; Marre, D.; Cabello, Á. Facial reanimation with gracilis muscle transfer neurotized to cross-facial nerve graft versus masseteric nerve: A comparative study using the FACIAL CLIMA evaluating system. *Plast. Reconstr. Surg.* **2013**, *131*, 1241–1252. [CrossRef]
9. Faris, C.; Heiser, A.; Hadlock, T.; Jowett, N. Free gracilis muscle transfer for smile reanimation after treatment for advanced parotid malignancy. *Head Neck* **2018**, *40*, 561–568. [CrossRef]
10. Collar, R.M.; Byrne, P.J.; Boahene, K.D.O. The subzygomatic triangle: Rapid, minimally invasive identification of the masseteric nerve for facial reanimation. *Plast. Reconstr. Surg.* **2013**, *132*, 183–188. [CrossRef]
11. Manktelow, R.T.; Tomat, L.R.; Zuker, R.M.; Chang, M. Smile reconstruction in adults with free muscle transfer innervated by the masseter motor nerve: Effectiveness and cerebral adaptation. *Plast. Reconstr. Surg.* **2006**, *118*, 885–899. [CrossRef]
12. Bitter, T.; Sorger, B.; Hesselmann, V.; Krug, B.; Lackner, K.; Guntinas-Lichius, O. Cortical representation sites of mimic movements after facial nerve reconstruction: A functional magnetic resonance imaging study. *Laryngoscope* **2011**, *121*, 699–706. [CrossRef]
13. Brown, M.C.; Holland, R.L.; Ironton, R. Nodal and terminal sprouting from motor nerves in fast and slow muscles of the mouse. *J. Physiol.* **1980**, *306*, 493–510. [CrossRef] [PubMed]
14. Diels, H. Current concepts in non-surgical facial nerve rehabilitation. In *The Facial Palsies. Complementary Approaches*; Lemma Publishers: Utrecht, The Netherlands, 2005; pp. 275–283.

15. Hontanilla, B.; Cabello, A. Spontaneity of smile after facial paralysis rehabilitation when using a non-facial donor nerve. *J. Craniomaxillofac. Surg.* **2016**, *44*, 1305–1309. [CrossRef]
16. Boahene, K.D. Dynamic muscle transfer in facial reanimation. *Facial Plast. Surg.* **2008**, *24*, 204–210. [CrossRef] [PubMed]
17. Bhama, P.K.; Weinberg, J.S.; Lindsay, R.W.; Hohman, M.H.; Cheney, M.L.; Hadlock, T.A. Objective outcomes analysis following microvascular gracilis transfer for facial reanimation: A review of 10 years' experience. *JAMA Facial Plast. Surg.* **2014**, *16*, 85–92. [CrossRef] [PubMed]
18. Stennert, E.; Limberg, C.H.; Frentrup, K.P. An index for paresis and defective healing–an easily applied method for objectively determining therapeutic results in facial paresis (author's transl). *Hno* **1977**, *25*, 238–245. [PubMed]
19. Lindsay, R.W.; Bhama, P.; Hadlock, T.A. Quality-of-life improvement after free gracilis muscle transfer for smile restoration in patients with facial paralysis. *JAMA Facial Plast. Surg.* **2014**, *16*, 419–424. [CrossRef]
20. Garcia, R.M.; Gosain, A.K.; Zenn, M.R.; Marcus, J.R. Early Postoperative Complications following Gracilis Free Muscle Transfer for Facial Reanimation: A Systematic Review and Pooled Data Analysis. *J. Reconstr. Microsurg.* **2015**, *31*, 558–564. [CrossRef]
21. Paletz, J.L.; Manktelow, R.T.; Chaban, R. The shape of a normal smile: Implications for facial paralysis reconstruction. *Plast. Reconstr. Surg.* **1994**, *93*, 784–789. [CrossRef]
22. Puls, W.C.; Jarvis, J.C.; Ruck, A.; Lehmann, T.; Guntinas-Lichius, O.; Volk, G.F. Surface electrical stimulation for facial paralysis is not harmful. *Muscle Nerve* **2020**, *61*, 347–353. [CrossRef]
23. Arnold, D.; Thielker, J.; Klingner, C.M.; Puls, W.C.; Misikire, W.; Guntinas-Lichius, O.; Volk, G.F. Selective Surface Electrostimulation of the Denervated Zygomaticus Muscle. *Diagnostics* **2021**, *11*, 188. [CrossRef]
24. Biglioli, F.; Colombo, V.; Tarabbia, F.; Autelitano, L.; Rabbiosi, D.; Colletti, G.; Giovanditto, F.; Battista, V.; Frigerio, A. Recovery of emotional smiling function in free-flap facial reanimation. *J. Oral Maxillofac. Surg.* **2012**, *70*, 2413–2418. [CrossRef] [PubMed]
25. Khan, M.N.; Rodriguez, L.G.; Pool, C.D.; Laitman, B.; Hernandez, C.; Erovic, B.M.; Teng, M.S.; Genden, E.M.; Miles, B.A. The versatility of the serratus anterior free flap in head and neck reconstruction. *Laryngoscope* **2017**, *127*, 568–573. [CrossRef] [PubMed]
26. Henry, F.P.; Leckenby, J.I.; Butler, D.P.; Grobbelaar, A.O. An algorithm to guide recipient vessel selection in cases of free functional muscle transfer for facial reanimation. *Arch. Plast. Surg.* **2014**, *41*, 716–721. [CrossRef] [PubMed]
27. Goyal, N.; Jowett, N.; Dwojak, S.; Cunane, M.B.; Zander, D.; Hadlock, T.A.; Emerick, K.S. Use of the submental vessels for free gracilis muscle transfer for smile reanimation. *Head Neck* **2016**, *38*, E2499–E2503. [CrossRef] [PubMed]
28. Lee, L.N.; Susarla, S.M.; Henstrom, D.K.; Hohman, M.H.; Durand, M.L.; Cheney, M.L.; Hadlock, T.A. Surgical site infections after gracilis free flap reconstruction for facial paralysis. *Otolaryngol. Head Neck Surg.* **2012**, *147*, 245–248. [CrossRef] [PubMed]

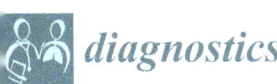

Article

Automatic Facial Palsy Diagnosis as a Classification Problem Using Regional Information Extracted from a Photograph

Gemma S. Parra-Dominguez [†], Carlos H. Garcia-Capulin *,[†] and Raul E. Sanchez-Yanez [†]

Department of Electronics Engineering, Universidad de Guanajuato DICIS, Salamanca 36885, Mexico; gs.parradominguez@ugto.mx (G.S.P.-D.); sanchezy@ugto.mx (R.E.S.-Y.)
* Correspondence: carlosg@ugto.mx
† These authors contributed equally to this work.

Abstract: The incapability to move the facial muscles is known as facial palsy, and it affects various abilities of the patient, for example, performing facial expressions. Recently, automatic approaches aiming to diagnose facial palsy using images and machine learning algorithms have emerged, focusing on providing an objective evaluation of the paralysis severity. This research proposes an approach to analyze and assess the lesion severity as a classification problem with three levels: healthy, slight, and strong palsy. The method explores the use of regional information, meaning that only certain areas of the face are of interest. Experiments carrying on multi-class classification tasks are performed using four different classifiers to validate a set of proposed hand-crafted features. After a set of experiments using this methodology on available image databases, great results are revealed (up to 95.61% of correct detection of palsy patients and 95.58% of correct assessment of the severity level). This perspective leads us to believe that the analysis of facial paralysis is possible with partial occlusions if face detection is accomplished and facial features are obtained adequately. The results also show that our methodology is suited to operate with other databases while attaining high performance, even though the image conditions are different and the participants do not perform equivalent facial expressions.

Keywords: clinical decision support systems; computerized assessment; facial palsy detection; facial paralysis diagnose; machine learning; medical diagnosis; medical screening; severity grading

1. Introduction

The inability to move the facial muscles on one or both sides is known as facial palsy or facial paralysis. This inability can be generated from nerve damage due to trauma, congenital conditions, or diseases like stroke, brain tumor, or Bell's palsy. Patients with facial palsy exhibit problems with speaking, blinking, swallowing saliva, eating, or communicating through natural facial expressions because of a noticeable drooping of facial capabilities. In general, the diagnosis by a clinician relies on a visual inspection of the patient's facial symmetry. The examination of facial palsy requires specific medical training to produce a diagnosis, and it could vary from practitioner to practitioner. This is a reason why, in recent years, automatic approaches based on computer vision and artificial intelligence have been emerging to provide an objective evaluation of the paralysis.

The wide variety of methodologies working with facial palsy found in the literature can be divided according to their primary task. For example, if the intention is to perform a binary classification to discriminate between healthy or unhealthy subjects (i.e., to detect facial palsy), or to perform a multi-class classification (i.e., to evaluate the level of paralysis). Automatic approaches based on computer vision and artificial intelligence that seek to detect facial palsy include the works in [1–6]. Binary classification can be performed with an objective other than detecting facial paralysis; for example, identifying the type of facial palsy that a patient suffers, as Barbosa et al. did in [2] when seeking to discriminate between peripheral palsy or central palsy.

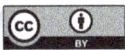

Automatic approaches aiming to assess the severity of facial palsy require a scale to measure the nerve damage. Those well-known scales are the House-Brackmann (HB), Sunnybrook, Yanagihara, FNGS 2.0, and eFACE. In detail, the grading scales split the facial nerve damage into a series of discrete levels according to some strict measures. Those measures are related to the symmetry of the face while displaying a neutral expression or showing a set of voluntary facial muscle movements; they are also associated with secondary features such as synkinesis [7]. Some authors, to start testing their algorithms, split the level of facial palsy into fewer degrees, for example: healthy, low, and high degrees of paralysis; and later report their findings [8–10].

Usually, automatic approaches are designed through handcrafted features and classifiers. Using a similar method, this research focuses on features computed from facial landmarks. As facial landmarks, we refer to the key points extracted using facial models on a face previously detected on an image. Many facial models (often referred to as shape predictors) are publicly available and can locate facial landmarks. Matthews and Baker introduced a 68-point facial model in [11], which is widely known and employed in the facial analysis field. However, few implementations fail in predicting those key points from persons who have facial palsy because the model was trained using imagery from healthy persons [12–14]. Recently, some authors have been working on improving the available shape predictors to extract facial landmarks in palsy patients accurately. Particularly relevant to our research is the model developed and released by Guarin et al. [15], which was trained using imagery of palsy patients.

The methodologies in [2,13,14,16] are based on handcrafted features extracted from facial landmarks and the use of a wide variety of classifiers. The asymmetry of the face is a core trait in those methodologies to diagnose facial palsy. Additionally, we wish to emphasize that the detection of facial paralysis was performed on proprietary databases with patients suffering from diverse levels of paralysis. To our knowledge those databases are unavailable to the research community, thus, a direct comparison of the performance is not possible. Some methodologies operate on specific facial gestures [13] and others require a set of movements to output a result [2,14,16]. Our proposed methodology is also based on handcrafted features, and they do not depend on a specific facial gesture to perform a classification task.

Diverse neural network structures have been applied to solve a variety of problems in the medical field [6,17–24]. Particularly, there are a few methodologies working with deep neural networks to evaluate facial palsy (e.g., [8,10,25–28]). Deep learning methods can improve the facial palsy detection rate, but their efficiency is limited by insufficient data and class imbalance, according to [28]. These methods automatically learn discriminative features, meaning that they do not compute handcrafted features but perform some preprocessing steps before training and evaluating the network. Due to the enormous amount of required data, geometric and color transformations, cropping, and resizing of the images are needed to increase the number of samples.

The methodologies in [10,26,28] are evaluated using the same facial palsy database; however, their experimental settings drastically differ in the testing method: leave-one-out protocol in [26], five-fold cross-validation in [10], and ten times repetitions in [28]. With this in mind, circumspect evaluations must be made when comparing performance. Both Hsu et al. [26] and Abayomi-Alli et al. [28] based their approach on well-known pre-trained networks with thousands of images. Particularly, Abayomi-Alli et al. extract 1000 deep features from a network's final layer, and those are fed to a classifier. Our proposed methodology requires a simpler classifier structure with few features and samples to perform a classification task.

The analysis of the human face in terms of symmetry/asymmetry is not a new topic, and there is plenty of literature about it [29,30]. We talk about the symmetry of a person's face knowing that we all are asymmetric. In other words, facial asymmetry responds to the fact that the left and right sides of our face showing no movement or while performing an expression are not identical. This asymmetry can be the result of various factors, including anatomical, neurological, physiological, pathological, psychological, and socio-cultural variables [29]. Usually, the growth and development of bones, nerves, and muscles should not produce new asymmetries.

We assume in this research that healthy faces have quite an identical left and right sides with a neutral expression, while the affected ones do not, allowing us to characterize the face of a palsy patient. In other words, a threshold value can be obtained using machine learning algorithms to determine to what extent the facial asymmetry is expected and where it is considered an unhealthy condition.

Our previous work in [6] introduced a system to detect facial palsy using 29 handcrafted geometrical features and a classifier based on neural networks. The objective was to classify face images into healthy and unhealthy regarding the severity of facial paralysis. There, the methodology operates on the assumption that facial paralysis can be characterized by locating levels of asymmetry in the face; if found, then it is said that the subject suffers from paralysis. The algorithm was evaluated in two different databases, obtaining a performance of 94.06% correct classification for the first database and 97.22% on the second one.

In this research, we also take the following perspectives in analyzing facial palsy. Some methodologies work with specific regions of the face (e.g., the mouth, the eyes, the forehead), and others extract helpful information from the entire face. Some approaches require a set of specific gestures to operate, and few need only one image to output a result. Finally, some methodologies perform binary discrimination between healthy and unhealthy subjects, and others evaluate different levels of paralysis based on a predefined clinical scale.

In this paper, we show that the framework introduced in [6] is independent of the facial gesture displayed by the person and that only one image is sufficient to output a result. We also show that our approach can perform multi-class classification tasks, and that the assessment of facial paralysis is possible with partial occlusions of the face if the analysis is executed on certain regions of the face. A performance analysis using four different classifiers is elaborated attaining excellent results to corroborate our features' validity in a wide range of situations.

The main contributions of this work are: (1) a methodology to design classifiers based on easy-to-compute features that do not require a set of facial gestures to output a result, (2) a framework to analyze facial palsy using information extracted from the entire face or from specific facial regions (the eyes or the mouth), (3) a performance analysis using four different classifiers with excellent results which could provide orientation in selecting the best classification approach, and (4) evaluations on publicly available databases.

The rest of this paper is organized as follows. Section 2 introduces the proposed methodology. Section 3 describes the databases employed in this research and introduces the experiments, findings, and discussion. Finally, concluding remarks are provided in Section 4.

2. Methodology

The framework of the facial palsy assessment system under consideration is depicted in Figure 1. The methodology starts with face detection within the input image, followed by the extraction of the facial landmarks using a shape predictor. The proposed 29 facial symmetry features are subsequently computed using these key points. Such features are fed to four different classifiers, trained depending on the system's goal. Detailed information will be provided next.

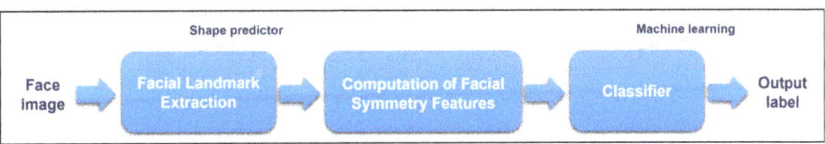

Figure 1. Framework of the proposed facial palsy assessment system.

2.1. Facial Landmark Extraction

The first step of the module is to detect the face within the image, which is achieved using the default face detector implemented in the open-source *dlib C++ Library*. That particular face detector was designed through a combination of a linear classifier with the Histogram of Oriented Gradients descriptor [31], an image pyramid, and a sliding-window detection scheme; further information can be found at [32]. The second step extracts the facial landmarks using the shape predictor proposed by Guarin et al. and introduced in [15]. The complete extraction process is as follows:

1. Transform the input image to gray levels.
2. (Optional) Resize the transformed image according to a scale factor (sf) of $sf = \frac{W}{nW}$, having $nW = 200$ and $nH = \frac{H}{sf}$. Where W and H refer to the width and height of the input image.
3. Detect the face rectangle on the smaller image.
4. (Optional) Re-scale the detected face rectangle to its original size using sf.
5. Extract the facial landmarks on the transformed image.
6. Store the predicted information for future processing.

Note that the shape predictor is a 68-point model, but only 51 points are of interest in this work. As sketched in Figure 2a, the 51 points are renumbered to ease the further calculation of attributes.

It is known that the head's tilt angle can influence the accuracy of the facial symmetry quantification [16]. Thus, a tilt correction is performed using two known points and a transformation matrix before computing any symmetry measure. The left corner of the left eye and the right corner of the right eye (points 10 and 19 as seen in Figure 2a) are set as known points. The complete process to correct the head's tilt angle is as follows:

1. Set as input data the eye-corner points.
2. Set the destination data on such points.
3. Calculate a transformation matrix T_f using the eye-corner points and the similarity transform approach.
4. (Optional) Transform the input image using the T_f matrix.
5. Rotate the predicted landmarks using the transformation T_f matrix.

The landmark rotation process can be performed following the multiplication of matrices stated in Equation (1)

$$\begin{pmatrix} Pir_x \\ Pir_y \end{pmatrix} = \begin{bmatrix} T_{f(1,1)} & T_{f(1,2)} & T_{f(1,3)} \\ T_{f(2,1)} & T_{f(2,2)} & T_{f(2,3)} \end{bmatrix} \begin{bmatrix} Pi_x \\ Pi_y \\ 1 \end{bmatrix} \quad (1)$$

2.2. Computation of Facial Symmetry Features

Computing and analyzing the asymmetry found within both sides of the face, left and right, has shown to be helpful when aiming to detect palsy regions; also, when seeking to evaluate the patient lesion's severity. The methodology mainly compares and quantifies the differences between both sides, specifically, the location and position of the facial organs (i.e., eyebrows, eyes, nose, and mouth). Initial tests led us to conclude that the regions of the eyebrows, eyes, and mouth provide meaningful information for this challenge, as reported by others [2,10,16,26]. Notice that some approaches require a set of images from the same subject performing specific gestures to operate (e.g., [2,4]), although it is strongly believed that the facial palsy assessment should not be conditioned to specific facial movements. Similar to [8], when a face image is loaded into our system, the facial gesture performed by the person does not need to be identified; therefore, the output of the system is a label obtained after an objective evaluation.

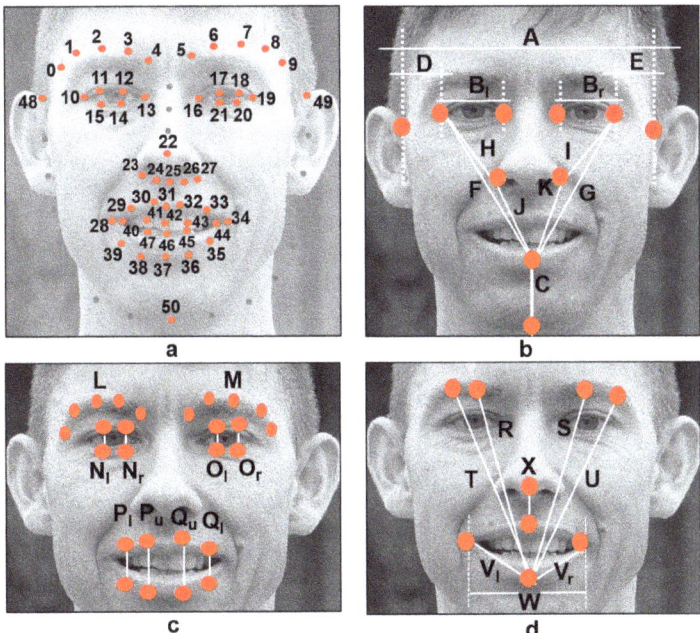

Figure 2. (a) The 51 key points inspired by the model proposed by Matthews and Baker [11]; (b–d) Facial distances to obtain spatial relations between facial landmarks [6].

In total, 28 distances and two average values are calculated using the predicted key points, as depicted in Figure 2b–d. Distances A to K are influenced by the research of Ostrofsky et al. [33], who focused on evaluating objective measures from face photographs with an intention other than facial paralysis detection, but they seem to be an excellent hint to represent the healthy human face. The rest of the distances (L to W), in Figure 2c,d, were found helpful in our previous work [6] to specifically provide independence from the facial movement executed by the subject.

In this research, we assume that a healthy face is pretty symmetric concerning the shape and position of the face elements, independently of the subject's facial gesture. If those elements are not symmetric, it is presumed that a grade of paralysis will be detected. Locating the affected side of the face is beyond the scope of this research.

The 29 proposed symmetry features are extracted using the 28 distances and the two average values introduced in Table 1. If additional information is required, please refer to Figure 2. Most of the computed distances provide ratios in the [0, 1] range, here 0 means somewhat asymmetric, and 1 means closer to a healthy face. Analogous ratios between the left and right sides are later compared, and the maximum value is selected; these are the features described as "Max" in Table 1. Other features were designed to represent the inclination between two key points, particularly in the eyebrows; these are the features described as "slope". It is expected for a healthy face to have a slope close to 0. Similarly, a few angles are computed between two key points. Again, it is expected for a healthy face to show an angle close to 0 (to be in a horizontal position), except for feature $f23$, which is expected to be vertical on a healthy subject. The features described as "ratio" reflect the asymmetry of the face; smaller values relate to a healthy subject and bigger values to an unhealthy one.

Table 1. Facial symmetry features, introduced by Parra-Dominguez et al. [6].

No.	Facial Region	Type	Formula
f0	Eyebrows	Angle	$\lvert\angle(P0, P9)\rvert$
f1	Eyebrows	Angle	$\lvert\angle(P2, P7)\rvert$
f2	Eyebrows	Angle	$\lvert\angle(P4, P5)\rvert$
f3	Eyebrows	Max.	$\max(L/M, M/L)$
f4	Eyebrows	Slope	$m(P0, P9)$
f5	Eyebrows	Slope	$m(P2, P7)$
f6	Eyebrows	Slope	$m(P4, P5)$
f7	Eyes	Angle	$\lvert\angle(P10, P19)\rvert$
f8	Eyes	Max.	$\max(B_l/B_r, B_r/B_l)$
f9	Eyes	Max.	$\max(D/E, E/D)$
f10	Eyes	Max.	$\max(H/I, I/H)$
f11	Eyes	Max.	$\max(N/O, O/N)$
f12	Eyes	Max.	$\max(N_l/O_r, O_r/N_l)$
f13	Eyes	Max.	$\max(N_r/O_l, O_l/N_r)$
f14	Mouth	Angle	$\lvert\angle(P28, P34)\rvert$
f15	Mouth	Max.	$\max(F/G, G/F)$
f16	Mouth	Max.	$\max(P_l/Q_l, Q_l/P_l)$
f17	Mouth	Max.	$\max(P_u/Q_u, Q_u/P_u)$
f18	Mouth	Max.	$\max(V_l/A, V_r/A)$
f19	Mouth	Max.	$\max(P_l/W, Q_l/W)$
f20	Mouth	Max.	$\max(P_u/W, Q_u/W)$
f21	Mouth	Max.	$\max(W_l/W, W_r/W)$
f22	Nose	Angle	$\lvert\angle(P23, P27)\rvert$
f23	Combined	Angle	$\lvert\angle(P22, P37)\rvert$
f24	Combined	Max.	$\max(J/K, K/J)$
f25	Combined	Max.	$\max(T/A, U/A)$
f26	Combined	Max.	$\max(R/A, S/A)$
f27	Combined	Ratio	C/A
f28	Combined	Ratio	X/A

In f3, L and M are the average height of all the left and right eyebrow points, respectively. In f11, $N = (N_l + N_r)/2$, similarly, $O = (O_l + O_r)/2$. In f19, f20, and f21, W is the distance shown in Figure 2d, and the perimeter values W_l and W_r are computed as $W_l = \overline{S}(P28, P29, P30, P31, P37, P38, P39)$ and $W_r = \overline{S}(P31, P32, P33, P34, P35, P36, P37)$.

The facial symmetry features are computed according to Equation (2) for the angle between key points, Equation (3) for the slope of key points, the Euclidean distance is used here and calculated according to Equation (4), and the perimeter of a closed shape is computed using Equation (5):

$$\angle(Pa, Pb) = \arctan 2(\triangle x, \triangle y) \times 180/\pi \qquad (2)$$

where $\triangle x = Pa_x - Pb_x$ and $\triangle y = Pa_y - Pb_y$.

$$m(Pa, Pb) = \left\lvert \frac{Pa_y - Pb_y}{Pa_x - Pb_x} \right\rvert \qquad (3)$$

$$d(Pa, Pb) = \sqrt{(Pa_x - Pb_x)^2 + (Pa_y - Pb_y)^2} \qquad (4)$$

$$\overline{S}(P_s, \ldots, P_e) = \sum_{x=s}^{l-1} d(P_x, P_x + 1) + d(P_s, P_e) \qquad (5)$$

where $\overline{S}$ is a closed shape, P_s is the start point, and P_e is the endpoint within the shape.

The use of regional information is explored in this paper to detect and evaluate facial paralysis. As mentioned before, a number of approaches extract meaningful information from the entire face; but it is also possible to extract useful information from specific areas of the face. Some of those areas are the eyebrows, the eyes, the nose, and the mouth, as shown in Figure 3. We refer to the features computed from those facial areas as regional information. Particularly in this research, experiments are carried out on the entire face, the eyes, and the mouth. Here, it is referred to as the entire face to the use of the 29 proposed symmetry features to execute classification tasks. For the eyes, only 19 features are considered and they correspond to features named as Eyebrows, Eyes, Nose, and Combined (only $f23$ and $f25$–$f27$) in Table 1. Consequently, the 15 features that correspond to the mouth are all features named Mouth, Nose, and Combined in Table 1.

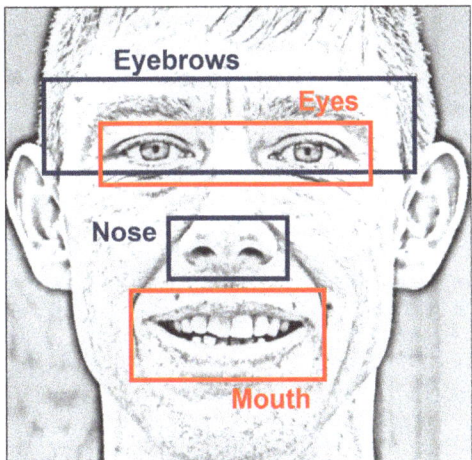

Figure 3. Example of a face image divided into four facial regions.

2.3. Classification

Our proposed classifiers were designed using the Waikato Environment for Knowledge Analysis (Weka) suite. Weka consists of a collection of machine learning algorithms for data mining tasks. It includes tools for data preparation, classification, regression, clustering, association rules mining, and visualization. In this work, four classifiers were configured based on the multi-layer perceptron (MLP), support vector machine (SVM), k-nearest-neighbor (KNN), and multinomial logistic regression (MNLR) methods. Depending on the implementation, each classifier requires specific parameters to operate, and those are optimized to reach the best performance. A list of some of those parameters is described in Table 2. More information concerning the Weka suite can be found at [34].

The Weka suite operates using Attribute-Relation File Format (arff) files, which are text files that describe a list of samples sharing a set of features and labels, for more information about how to create them, refer to [35]. In this work, after computing the data set composed of features extracted from healthy and palsy patients, an arff file for each training and testing set was created by running an easy-to-implement script. Then the files are loaded into Weka, and the training process begins, ending with the evaluation process. Further details on the tests and results are provided next.

Table 2. Required parameters to operate the classifier in the Weka suite, according to [34].

Method	Parameters	Weka Function
MLP	Learning rate (L), momentum (M), training time (N), number of neurons in the hidden layers (H), and seed (S)	MultilayerPerceptron
SVM	Cost (C), gamma (G), kernel type	LibSVM
KNN	Number of neighbors (KNN) and distance function (A)	IBk
MNLR	Ridge (R)	Logistic

In Weka, the parameter N of MLP refers to the number of epochs to train through and the nodes in the network are all sigmoid. Additionally, the radial basis function (RBF) kernel was used in all experiments using SVM and only one neighbor was set for the KNN classifier.

3. Results and Discussion

A few methodologies in the literature look to assess facial paralysis in an image. Then, it seems relevant to mention that collaborating with the research community has been complicated due to the unavailability of public databases, mainly because of the need of preserving the patient's privacy. This scenario encouraged us to evaluate our system on a database that is publicly available. As stated previously, this research seeks to expand our previous methodology to perform the tasks of detection and assessment of facial palsy regions. In this work, three experiments were executed to evaluate the performance of four different classification methods. The results and findings are discussed in the following paragraphs.

Comments on the database where images of palsy patients were extracted are given now. The YouTube Facial Palsy (YFP) database is an image collection provided by Hsu et al. [9]. The YFP database is a compilation of 32 videos from 21 patients obtained from YouTube; 10 additional patients in a second release were included. The patient talks to the camera in each video, and the facial expression variation across time is recorded. Each video was converted into an image sequence at 6 FPS, yielding almost 3000 images. Three independent clinicians labeled the palsy regions in each frame; the junction of the independently cropped areas is considered the ground truth. The authors also provided additional labels to classify the intensity exhibited in each palsy region. It is our understanding that the authors in [9] determined these intensity labels; they did not declare that the intensity label was approved by a clinician, which could lead to discrepancies in the classification results among methodologies. The YFP is available upon request at [36].

The Extended Cohn-Kanade (CK+) database distribution, a well-known database in the research community to prototype and benchmark systems for the automated detection of facial expression [37], was also employed. The CK+ database collects 593 sequences across 123 subjects, close to 10,800 images, and all sequences go from a neutral face to a peak expression. The CK+ database is included in this work, with the YFP database, to make our methodology robust against expression variation as suggested in [9,10]. The unhealthy samples came from the YFP database and the healthy subjects from the CK+.

Widely known evaluation metrics are computed to measure the performance of each classifier. These are accuracy, recall (or true positive rate), precision, F1 score, true negative rate, false negative rate, and false positive rate which are calculated according to Equations (6)–(12), respectively.

$$Acc = \frac{TP + TN}{TP + TN + FP + FN} \qquad (6)$$

$$Rec = \frac{TP}{TP + FN} \qquad (7)$$

$$Prec = \frac{TP}{TP + FP} \qquad (8)$$

$$F1s = \frac{2 \times TP}{2 \times TP + FP + FN} \qquad (9)$$

$$TNR = \frac{TN}{TN + FP} \qquad (10)$$

$$FNR = \frac{FN}{FN + TP} \qquad (11)$$

$$FPR = \frac{FP}{FP + TN} \qquad (12)$$

where TP is short for true positives, TN for true negatives, FP for false positives, and FN for false negatives.

The 5-fold cross-validation protocol was adopted to test the model accuracy for each classification task. Such protocol allows us to test on unseen samples, reducing the possibility of over-fitting to previously seen ones. This cross-validation strategy splits the data set into five subsets. Every subset is preserved as validation data, and the other four are used as training data, ensuring that the test data is untouched in each experiment occurrence. The experiment is repeated five times, where each subset has the same probability for validation. The accumulation of correct classified samples measures the performance.

3.1. Palsy Region Detection

The first experiments are focused on detecting facial palsy, in other words, on classifying the input data as healthy or unhealthy. It is called palsy region detection because those particular algorithms analyze specific facial regions. Here, the experiments evaluate our methodology using regional information, but our initial proposal is to inspect the whole face using our symmetry features. Three tests were performed: (1) the detection of palsy using 29 features, (2) the detection of palsy in the eyes, and (3) the detection of palsy in the mouth. As described earlier, the regional information for the eyes correspond to features named as Eyebrows, Eyes, Nose, and Combined (only f23 and f25–f27) in Table 1. Similarly, the regional information for the mouth corresponds to all features, except those named as Eyebrows and Eyes features in Table 1.

In general, the data set is composed of 19 palsy patients and 19 healthy subjects. The palsy patients are subjects 1, 5, 6, 7, 11, 12, 13, 14, 15, 19, 20, 21, 23, 24, 25, 28, 29, 30, and 31 from the YFP database. Patients with less than 20 images and patients with facial occlusions were excluded. The healthy subjects belong to the S022, S026, S028, S034, S042, S046, S050, S054, S057, S102, S105, S124, S130, S131, S132, S133, S134, S135, and S136 folders in the CK+ collection.

The data set for the first experiment comprises 20 images from each of the 38 participants (760 images in total); this arrangement is expected to have the same amount of healthy and palsy samples, making it a balanced data set for the experiment. Notice that the healthy subjects are labeled as class 0 and the palsy subjects as class 1. For this experiment, the classifiers were configured as described in Table 3. The experiment using 5-fold cross-validation was repeated 10 times, and the average performance is shown in Table 4, for the three tests.

Table 3. First experiment: classifiers' configuration.

Method	Parameters
MLP	$L = 0.2045, M = 0.1909, H = 59, N = 5000, S = 0$
SVM	$C = 1000, G = \{0.1, 0.001, 0.01\}$ *, kernel type = RBF
KNN	$KNN = 1, A =$ Euclidean distance
MNLR	$R = 1 \times 10^{-8}$

* Refers to the gamma value for the face, eyes, and mouth evaluation, respectively.

Table 4. Results of the detection of palsy regions on the criteria of accuracy.

Classifier	Face	Eyes	Mouth
MLP	95.03 ± 1.69%	92.86 ± 1.99%	92.98 ± 2.13%
SVM	95.61 ± 1.40%	93.42 ± 1.84%	90.93 ± 2.49%
KNN	92.34 ± 1.80%	89.33 ± 2.24%	91.28 ± 2.21%
MNLR	94.24 ± 1.60%	92.16 ± 1.99%	91.07 ± 2.35%

Great results are obtained for the MLP and SVM classifiers, 95.03% and 95.61%, respectively. Few samples were required during the training phase compared to other approaches that required thousands of images to output a label. Good results are also reached using only regional features, in the eye and the mouth, 93.42% and 92.98%, respectively. Still, the entire face analysis is better than focusing on a single region when discriminating between healthy and unhealthy subjects.

The confusion matrix of this experiment using the entire face and SVM is depicted in Figure 4a, and the system's average accuracy is 95.61%, recall 95.63%, precision 95.61% and F1-score 95.62%. The confusion matrix analyzing the eyes with SVM is depicted in Figure 4b, and the system's average accuracy is 93.42%, recall 94.47%, precision 92.55% and F1-score 93.50%. Finally, the confusion matrix analyzing the eyes with MLP is depicted in Figure 4c, and the system's average accuracy is 92.98%, recall 94.63%, precision 91.64% and F1-score 93.11%.

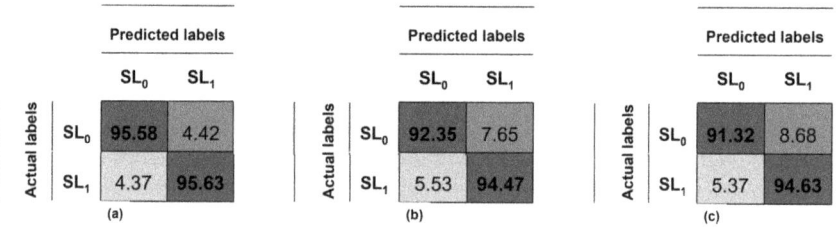

Figure 4. Confusion matrix of the detection of the palsy: (**a**) on the entire face, (**b**) on the eyes region and (**c**) on the mouth region.

Additional performance results for the experiments are provided on Table 5. For our methodology, the true negative rate (TNR) reflects the number of healthy subjects detected as normal participants; while the true positive rate (TPR) shows the number of palsy patients detected as unhealthy subjects. Great results are achieved using the SVM classifier: 95.59% and 95.63% for the face, 92.35% and 94.47% for the eyes. On the other hand, the false negative and false positive rates are expected to be as lower as possible because both of them represent a wrong diagnosis. Good results are obtained for this metric: 4.37% and 4.41% for the face, 5.53% and 7.65% for the eyes. Similarly, good results are reached for the mouth using the MLP classifier, 91.32% and 94.63% of true detection rates; and 5.37% and 8.68% of false detection rates.

Table 5. Performance results for the detection of palsy regions.

Region	Classifier	TNR	FNR	TPR	FPR
Face	SVM	95.59 ± 2.28%	4.37 ± 2.05%	95.63 ± 2.05%	4.41 ± 2.28%
Eyes	SVM	92.35 ± 3.11%	5.53 ± 2.81%	94.47 ± 2.81%	7.65 ± 3.11%
Mouth	MLP	91.32 ± 3.51%	5.37 ± 2.85%	94.63 ± 2.85%	8.68 ± 3.51%

Although out of the scope of this work, those scores using either the eye or mouth information lead us to believe that we can use these features to detect facial palsy on images with partial occlusions. If face detection is achieved and landmarks are predicted adequately, an analysis to detect facial palsy might be possible. In other words, our analysis allows us to determine to what extent regional information is needed to diagnose the severity of the lesion with satisfactory results.

3.2. Prediction of Two Palsy Levels

The second experiment seeks to distinguish between two levels of facial palsy. As stated by Hsu et al. [9], these levels are slight (or low-intensity) and strong (or high-intensity) facial palsy. The authors provided labels for the mouth and the eyes regions; there might be a case where the intensity is not the same for both regions, then a separate analysis is required. The data set is composed of 19 patients from the YFP database and is now divided into class SL_1 (low-intensity) and class SL_2 (high-intensity). After preliminary tests, it was found that 40 images per patient were adequate to train the classifier, but for those who did not have enough images, only 20 were employed. To improve the learning process, a data augmentation was performed as suggested in [1,16]. This process consisted of rotating in two opposite directions the palsy images to increase the amount of available data. This augmentation also allows us to verify that the algorithm is invariant to rotation, as stated in Section 2.1. This experiment is divided into two tests (1) using the 29 proposed features and (2) using regional information (19 features for the eyes and 15 features for the mouth).

The data distribution for this experiment is described in Table 6. There, to evaluate the level of paralysis in the eyes, 208 low-intensity and 472 high-intensity images are included. After data augmentation, the data set is formed by 624 low-intensity and 1416 high-intensity samples (2040 images in total). Similarly, to evaluate the level of paralysis in the mouth, 141 low-intensity and 539 high-intensity images are included. After data augmentation, the data set is formed by 423 low-intensity and 1617 high-intensity samples (2040 images in total).

Table 6. Data distribution for the prediction of two palsy levels.

Test	Total of Images	Data Distribution
Eyes region	680	Original data: 208 low-intensity and 472 high-intensity samples
	2040	Augmented data: 624 low-intensity and 1416 high-intensity samples
Mouth region	680	Original data: 141 low-intensity and 539 high-intensity samples
	2040	Augmented data: 423 low-intensity and 1617 high-intensity samples

For the first test, the configuration of the classifiers is described in Table 7. A 5-fold cross-validation was performed and repeated 10 times, and the average performance is shown in Table 8 for both regions. Great results are obtained assessing the eyes region, up to 95.05% using SVM. Similarly, good results are reached for the mouth area, 92.69%. In this task, the KNN classifier reached better results than the MLP for both cases. Still, the proposed MLP yielded good results using few samples, compared to other published deep learning approaches that require thousands of images and complex neural network structures.

For the second test, the configuration of the classifiers is described in Table 9. Again a 5-fold cross-validation repeated 10 times was performed, and the average performance is shown in Table 10 for both regions using fewer features. It was expected a lower performance because the information feed to the classifiers was decreased; still, good performance (more than 90%) was achieved using SVM. A slight increase in performance is observed when using the information from the mouth region. This evaluation leads us to believe that a classification of the palsy intensity is possible to a certain degree, in partial occlusions of the face.

Table 7. Second experiment: classifiers' configuration for the first test.

Method	Parameters
MLP	$L = 0.2045, M = 0.1909, H = 59, N = \{500, 2000\}$ *, $S = \{2, 37\}$ *
SVM	$C = 1000, G = 1.0$, kernel type = RBF
KNN	$KNN = 1, A =$ Manhattan distance
MNLR	$R = 1 \times 10^{-8}$

* Refers to the values for the eyes and mouth evaluation, respectively.

Table 8. Results on the prediction of two palsy levels on the criteria of accuracy using the 29 symmetry features.

Classifier	Eyes	Mouth
MLP	92.39 ± 1.23%	90.20 ± 1.27%
SVM	95.05 ± 1.14%	92.69 ± 1.01%
KNN	93.54 ± 1.24%	92.14 ± 1.16%
MNLR	82.96 ± 1.83%	81.09 ± 1.47%

Table 9. Second experiment: classifiers' configuration for the second test.

Method	Parameters
MLP	$L = 0.2045, M = 0.1909, H = 59, N = \{1000, 500\}$ *, $S = \{87, 7\}$ *
SVM	$C = 10, G = 1.0$, kernel type = RBF
KNN	$KNN = 1, A =$ Manhattan distance
MNLR	$R = 1 \times 10^{-8}$

* Refers to the values for the eyes and mouth evaluation, respectively.

Table 10. Results on the prediction of two palsy levels on the criteria of accuracy using regional information.

Classifier	Eyes	Mouth
MLP	88.75 ± 1.87%	89.60 ± 1.27%
SVM	91.12 ± 1.57%	93.29 ± 1.22%
KNN	89.99 ± 1.54%	91.70 ± 0.94%
MNLR	79.97 ± 1.97%	80.15 ± 1.13%

3.3. Prediction of Three Palsy Levels

The goal of assessing the severity of the lesion is to determine how diminished the facial nerve function is. It can be evaluated once the palsy has been detected or evaluated at the same time. For the third experiment, the intensity labels provided by Hsu et al. [9] were also used. As previously mentioned, the authors offer labels for the mouth and the eyes' regions independently, and there might be a case where the intensity label is not the same for both regions. The data set is now divided into class SL_0 (healthy), class SL_1 (slight palsy or low-intensity), and class SL_2 (strong palsy or high-intensity). In Figure 5, a sample of healthy subjects and patients who have facial palsy is introduced. Specifically, the images show the two facial palsy regions that are of interest in this work: the eyes and mouth.

This experiment is also divided into two tests (1) using the 29 proposed features and (2) using regional information (19 features for the eyes and 15 features for the mouth). The data set is composed of 19 patients from the YFP database and 19 participants from the CK+ database. In this case, 40 images per subject were used; for those who did not have enough images, only 20 were employed. Once more, the same data augmentation process was performed to provide enough information to the classifiers, increasing the amount of data and verifying that the methodology is rotation invariant.

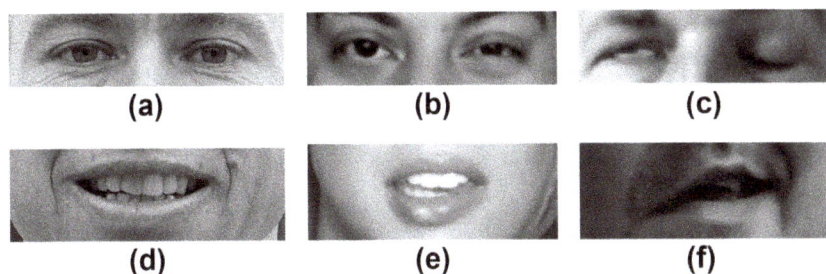

Figure 5. Facial analysis: (**a**) healthy eyes, (**b**) slight palsy and (**c**) strong palsy eyes; (**d**) healthy mouth, (**e**) slight palsy, and (**f**) strong palsy mouth. Palsy images were obtained from [9].

The data distribution is described in Table 11. For the eyes' region, 740 healthy, 208 low-intensity, and 472 high-intensity samples are included; it is easy to observe that the classes are unbalanced and that there are few examples for the class SL_1. After augmenting the samples, 4260 images compose the training set with 2220 healthy, 624 low-intensity, and 1416 high-intensity samples. For the mouth region, 740 healthy samples, 141 low-intensity, and 539 high-intensity samples are included; again, there are fewer examples for the class SL_1. After augmenting the samples, 4260 images compose the training set with 2220 healthy, 423 low-intensity, and 1617 high-intensity samples. In both tests, the classes remained unbalanced, but after several evaluations, this data distribution provided the best results.

Table 11. Data distribution for the prediction of three palsy levels.

Test	Total of Images	Data Distribution
Eyes region	1420	Original data: 740 healthy, 208 low-intensity and 472 high-intensity samples
	4260	Augmented data: 2220 healthy, 624 low-intensity and 1416 high-intensity samples
Mouth region	1420	Original data: 740 healthy, 141 low-intensity and 539 high-intensity samples
	4260	Augmented data: 2220 healthy, 423 low-intensity and 1617 high-intensity samples

The configuration of the classifiers is described in Table 12. The experiment using 5-fold cross-validation was repeated 10 times, and the average performance is shown in Table 13, for both regions. Great results are obtained assessing the eyes region, up to 95.58% using SVM. Similarly, good results are reached for the mouth area, 94.44%. In both cases, the proposed MLP yielded similar results using few samples, compared to other deep learning strategies that require thousands of samples and complex neural network structures.

Table 12. Third experiment: classifiers' configuration for the first test.

Method	Parameters
MLP	$L = 0.2045, M = 0.1909, H = 59, N = \{1000, 7000\}$ *, $S = \{18, 25\}$ *
SVM	$C = \{10, 1000\}$ *, $G = 1.0$, kernel type = RBF
KNN	$KNN = 1, A =$ Manhattan distance
MNLR	$R = 1 \times 10^{-8}$

* Refers to the values for the eyes and mouth evaluation, respectively.

Table 13. Results on the palsy lesion assessment on the criteria of accuracy using the 29 symmetry features.

Classifier	Eyes	Mouth
MLP	93.67 ± 0.94%	92.77 ± 0.87%
SVM	95.58 ± 0.71%	94.44 ± 0.63%
KNN	93.21 ± 0.80%	92.94 ± 0.80%
MNLR	86.48 ± 0.82%	85.95 ± 0.77%

For the second test, the configuration of the classifiers is described in Table 14. Again a 5-fold cross-validation was performed and repeated 10 times, and the average performance is shown in Table 15 for both regions using fewer features. It was expected a lower performance because the information fed to the classifiers was decreased; still, good performance, 92.08% and 93.95% were achieved using SVM. Once more, this evaluation leads us to believe that a classification of the palsy intensity is possible to a certain degree, in partial occlusions of the face.

Table 14. Third experiment: classifiers' configuration for the second test.

Method	Parameters
MLP	$L = 0.2045, M = 0.1909, H = 59, N = \{4000, 7000\}$ *, $S = \{18, 25\}$ *
SVM	$C = 10, G = 1.0$, kernel type = RBF
KNN	$KNN = 1, A = $ {Manhattan, Euclidean distance}
MNLR	$R = 1 \times 10^{-8}$

* Refers to the values for the eyes and mouth evaluation, respectively.

Table 15. Results on the palsy lesion assessment on the criteria of accuracy using regional information.

Classifier	Eyes	Mouth
MLP	89.63 ± 1.04%	91.91 ± 0.94%
SVM	92.08 ± 0.79%	93.95 ± 0.62%
KNN	89.24 ± 0.92%	92.08 ± 0.83%
MNLR	83.07 ± 1.07%	84.30 ± 0.76%

4. Conclusions

A methodology to assess facial paralysis in an image was proposed. It is assumed that facial palsy can be interpreted as a problem of asymmetry levels between the elements of the face, particularly the eyebrows, eyes, and mouth. The proposed assessment system consists of 29 facial symmetry features extracted from predicted landmarks and a classifier that provides a label as an output. Four different classifiers were evaluated in three experiments to validate our methodology. Those experiments seek to detect facial palsy, discriminate among two levels of the palsy, and assess the lesion's severity among three levels of palsy. The best results were achieved using SVM, but a similar performance with a slight decrease is obtained using the multi-layer perceptron approach. After the evaluations, it was found that dividing the face into specific regions is convenient to detect and assess the paralysis with fewer features. This feature reduction leads us to believe that the analysis of facial paralysis is possible with partial occlusions of the face, as long as face detection is achieved, and landmarks are predicted adequately.

To validate the proposed methodology, tests were performed on publicly available image databases, the YouTube Facial Palsy (YFP) with 21 participants with facial palsy, and the CK+ with 123 healthy subjects. In the first classification task, binary discrimination between healthy and unhealthy subjects, the proposed system achieved the highest accuracy of 95.61% after evaluating using the 5-fold cross-validation protocol. In a second task, a binary classification to detect the intensity of the facial palsy (low-intensity vs. high-intensity), the system achieved the highest accuracy of 95.05% in the eyes and 93.29% in the mouth region. Finally, in a third task to classify the severity of the damage (healthy, low-intensity, and high-intensity), the system achieved the highest accuracy of 95.58% for the eyes and 94.44% for the mouth.

It has been noted that evaluating facial paralysis using symmetry/asymmetry values is risky because the human face is not identical concerning its left and right sides. Then, to thoroughly verify the usefulness of our algorithm in clinical practice, a much larger sample of healthy controls with different degrees of facial asymmetry (not caused by facial palsy) is needed. Achieving this monumental task would require a specific database of healthy participants (i.e., showing no facial palsy of any kind) and a multidisciplinary team of experts to design a grading scale of healthy asymmetry, to calculate how asymmetric is the subject's face according to it, and to label each participant's image manually. To the best of our knowledge, no such data set is available for the research community.

Future work would include additional evaluations on available databases, with annotated data, of palsy patients and healthy controls. The design of a mobile application to diagnose facial palsy at home is also desirable to improve the rate of early diagnosis. Furthermore, developing an application to easily monitor the treatment and improvement of the patient would represent a milestone.

To conclude, the accomplished results show that the proposed methodology to design classifiers can be adapted to other data sets with outstanding results. It is a methodology that is easy to replicate compared to the other complex systems and achieves similar results for detecting and evaluating facial paralysis. Finally, the proposed classifiers require fewer samples in the training stage compared to different approaches based on deep neural networks. The code to compute the 29 facial symmetry features and the trained models are available upon request; notice that the image databases must be requested from the rightful owners at [36,37].

Author Contributions: Conceptualization, G.S.P.-D., C.H.G.-C. and R.E.S.-Y.; formal analysis, R.E.S.-Y. and C.H.G.-C.; investigation, G.S.P.-D.; methodology, G.S.P.-D., R.E.S.-Y. and C.H.G.-C.; project administration, C.H.G.-C. and R.E.S.-Y.; supervision, C.H.G.-C.; validation G.S.P.-D., R.E.S.-Y. and C.H.G.-C.; writing—original draft, G.S.P.-D.; writing—review and editing, G.S.P.-D., R.E.S.-Y. and C.H.G.-C. All authors have read and agreed to the published version of the manuscript.

Funding: This research received funding from the National Council of Science and Technology of Mexico (CONACYT) through the scholarship 302076.

Institutional Review Board Statement: Not applicable.

Informed Consent Statement: Not applicable.

Data Availability Statement: Not applicable.

Acknowledgments: The authors wish to thank the National Council of Science and Technology of Mexico (CONACYT) for the support provided to this research through the scholarship 302076.

Conflicts of Interest: The authors declare no conflict of interest.

References

1. Kim, H.S.; Kim, S.Y.; Kim, Y.H.; Park, K.S. A smartphone-based automatic diagnosis system for facial nerve palsy. *Sensors* **2015**, *15*, 26756–26768. [CrossRef] [PubMed]
2. Barbosa, J.; Lee, K.; Lee, S.; Lodhi, B.; Cho, J.G.; Seo, W.K.; Kang, J. Efficient quantitative assessment of facial paralysis using iris segmentation and active contour-based key points detection with hybrid classifier. *BMC Med. Imaging* **2016**, *16*, 23. [CrossRef] [PubMed]
3. Song, A.; Xu, G.; Ding, X.; Song, J.; Xu, G.; Zhang, W. Assessment for facial nerve paralysis based on facial asymmetry. *Australas. Phys. Eng. Sci. Med.* **2017**, *40*, 851–860. [CrossRef]
4. Barbosa, J.; Seo, W.K.; Kang, J. paraFaceTest: An ensemble of regression tree-based facial features extraction for efficient facial paralysis classification. *BMC Med. Imaging* **2019**, *19*, 30. [CrossRef]
5. Zhuang, Y.; McDonald, M.; Uribe, O.; Yin, X.; Parikh, D.; Southerland, A.M.; Rohde, G.K. Facial Weakness Analysis and Quantification of Static Images. *IEEE J. Biomed. Health Inform.* **2020**, *24*, 2260–2267. [CrossRef]

6. Parra-Dominguez, G.S.; Sanchez-Yanez, R.E.; Garcia-Capulin, C.H. Facial Paralysis Detection on Images Using Key Point Analysis. *Appl. Sci.* **2021**, *11*, 2435. [CrossRef]
7. Thevenot, J.; López, M.B.; Hadid, A. A survey on computer vision for assistive medical diagnosis from faces. *IEEE J. Biomed. Health Inform.* **2018**, *22*, 1497–1511. [CrossRef]
8. Song, A.; Wu, Z.; Ding, X.; Hu, Q.; Di, X. Neurologist Standard Classification of Facial Nerve Paralysis with Deep Neural Networks. *Future Internet* **2018**, *10*, 111. [CrossRef]
9. Hsu, G.S.J.; Kang, J.H.; Huang, W.F. Deep Hierarchical Network With Line Segment Learning for Quantitative Analysis of Facial Palsy. *IEEE Access* **2019**, *7*, 4833–4842. [CrossRef]
10. Liu, X.; Xia, Y.; Yu, H.; Dong, J.; Jian, M.; Pham, T.D. Region Based Parallel Hierarchy Convolutional Neural Network for Automatic Facial Nerve Paralysis Evaluation. *IEEE Trans. Neural Syst. Rehabil. Eng.* **2020**, *28*, 2325–2332. [CrossRef]
11. Matthews, I.; Baker, S. Active appearance models revisited. *Int. J. Comput. Vis.* **2004**, *60*, 135–164. [CrossRef]
12. Guarin, D.L.; Dusseldorp, J.; Hadlock, T.A.; Jowett, N. A machine learning approach for automated facial measurements in facial palsy. *JAMA Facial Plast. Surg.* **2018**, *20*, 335–337. [CrossRef]
13. Jiang, C.; Wu, J.; Zhong, W.; Wei, M.; Tong, J.; Yu, H.; Wang, L. Automatic facial paralysis assessment via computational image analysis. *J. Healthc. Eng.* **2020**, *2020*, 2398542. [CrossRef]
14. Wang, T.; Zhang, S.; Yu, H.; Dong, J.; Liu, L.A. Automatic evaluation of the degree of facial nerve paralysis. *Multimed. Tools Appl.* **2016**, *75*, 11893–11908. [CrossRef]
15. Guarin, D.L.; Yunusova, Y.; Taati, B.; Dusseldorp, J.R.; Mohan, S.; Tavares, J.; van Veen, M.M.; Fortier, E.; Hadlock, T.A.; Jowett, N. Toward an automatic system for computer-aided assessment in facial palsy. *Facial Plast. Surg. Aesthetic Med.* **2020**, *22*, 42–49. [CrossRef]
16. Guo, Z.; Dan, G.; Xiang, J.; Wang, J.; Yang, W.; Ding, H.; Deussen, O.; Zhou, Y. An unobtrusive computerized assessment framework for unilateral peripheral facial paralysis. *IEEE J. Biomed. Health Inform.* **2018**, *22*, 835–841. [CrossRef]
17. Azar, A.T. Fast neural network learning algorithms for medical applications. *Neural Comput. Appl.* **2013**, *23*, 1019–1034. [CrossRef]
18. Kabir, H.M.D.; Khosravi, A.; Hosen, M.A.; Nahavandi, S. Neural Network-Based Uncertainty Quantification: A Survey of Methodologies and Applications. *IEEE Access* **2018**, *6*, 36218–36234. [CrossRef]
19. Albu, A.; Precup, R.E.; Teban, T.A. Results and Challenges of Artificial Neural Networks used for Decision-Making and Control in Medical Applications. *Mech. Eng.* **2019**, *17*, 285–308. [CrossRef]
20. Smys, S.; Chen, J.I.Z.; Shakya, S. Survey on Neural Network Architectures with Deep Learning. *J. Soft Comput. Paradig. (JSCP)* **2020**, *2*, 186–194. [CrossRef]
21. Izonin, I.; Tkachenko, R.; Gregus, M.; Ryvak, L.; Kulyk, V.; Chopyak, V. Hybrid Classifier via PNN-based Dimensionality Reduction Approach for Biomedical Engineering Task. *Procedia Comput. Sci.* **2021**, *191*, 230–237 [CrossRef]
22. Parra-Dominguez, G.S.; Sanchez-Yanez, R.E.; Garcia-Capulin, C.H. Towards Facial Gesture Recognition in Photographs of Patients with Facial Palsy. *Healthcare* **2022**, *10*, 659. [CrossRef]
23. Izonin, I.; Tkachenko, R.; Duriagina, Z.; Shakhovska, N.; Kovtun, V.; Lotoshynska, N. Smart Web Service of Ti-Based Alloy's Quality Evaluation for Medical Implants Manufacturing. *Appl. Sci.* **2022**, *12*, 5238. [CrossRef]
24. Taran, V.; Gordienko, Y.; Rokovyi, O.; Alienin, O.; Kochura, Y.; Stirenko, S. Edge Intelligence for Medical Applications Under Field Conditions. In *Advances in Artificial Systems for Logistics Engineering*; Hu, Z., Zhang, Q., Petoukhov, S., He, M., Eds.; Springer International Publishing: Cham, Switzerland, 2022; pp. 71–80.
25. Guo, Z.; Shen, M.; Duan, L.; Zhou, Y.; Xiang, J.; Ding, H.; Chen, S.; Deussen, O.; Dan, G. Deep assessment process: Objective assessment process for unilateral peripheral facial paralysis via deep convolutional neural network. In Proceedings of the 2017 IEEE 14th International Symposium on Biomedical Imaging (ISBI 2017), Melbourne, Australia, 18–21 April 2017 ; pp. 135–138. [CrossRef]
26. Hsu, G.S.J.; Huang, W.F.; Kang, J.H. Hierarchical network for facial palsy detection. In Proceedings of the 2018 IEEE/CVF Conference on Computer Vision and Pattern Recognition Workshops (CVPRW), Salt Lake City, UT, USA, 18–22 June 2018; pp. 693–699. [CrossRef]
27. Sajid, M.; Shafique, T.; Baig, M.J.A.; Riaz, I.; Amin, S.; Manzoor, S. Automatic grading of palsy using asymmetrical facial features: A study complemented by new solutions. *Symmetry* **2018**, *10*, 242. [CrossRef]
28. Abayomi-Alli, O.O.; Damaševičius, R.; Maskeliūnas, R.; Misra, S. Few-Shot Learning with a Novel Voronoi Tessellation-Based Image Augmentation Method for Facial Palsy Detection. *Electronics* **2021**, *10*, 978. [CrossRef]
29. Borod, J.C.; van Gelder, R.S. INTRODUCTION. *Int. J. Psychol.* **1990**, *25*, 135–139. [CrossRef]
30. Codari, M.; Pucciarelli, V.; Stangoni, F.; Zago, M.; Tarabbia, F.; Biglioli, F.; Sforza, C. Facial thirds–based evaluation of facial asymmetry using stereophotogrammetric devices: Application to facial palsy subjects. *J. -Cranio-Maxillofac. Surg.* **2017**, *45*, 76–81. [CrossRef] [PubMed]
31. Dalal, N.; Triggs, B. Histograms of oriented gradients for human detection. In Proceedings of the 2005 IEEE Computer Society Conference on Computer Vision and Pattern Recognition (CVPR'05), San Diego, CA, USA, 20–25 June 2005; Volume 1, pp. 886–893. [CrossRef]
32. King, D.E. Dlib-ml: A Machine Learning Toolkit. *J. Mach. Learn. Res.* **2009**, *10*, 1755–1758.
33. Ostrofsky, J.; Cohen, D.J.; Kozbelt, A. Objective versus subjective measures of face-drawing accuracy and their relations with perceptual constancies. *Psychol. Aesthetics Creat. Arts* **2014**, *8*, 486–497. [CrossRef]

34. Witten, I.H.; Frank, E.; Hall, M.A. *Data Mining: Practical Machine Learning Tools and Techniques*, 3rd ed.; Morgan Kaufmann: Burlington, MA, USA, 2011.
35. Paynter, G. Attribute-Relation File Format (ARFF). 2002. Available online: https://www.cs.waikato.ac.nz/ml/weka/arff.html (accessed on 22 March 2021).
36. Hsu, G.S. YouTube Facial Palsy (YFP) Database. 2020. Available online: https://sites.google.com/view/yfp-database/ (accessed on 21 January 2021).
37. Lucey, P.; Cohn, J.F.; Kanade, T.; Saragih, J.; Ambadar, Z.; Matthews, I. The Extended Cohn-Kanade Dataset (CK+): A complete dataset for action unit and emotion-specified expression. In Proceedings of the 2010 IEEE Computer Society Conference on Computer Vision and Pattern Recognition—Workshops, San Francisco, CA, USA, 13–18 June 2010; pp. 94–101. [CrossRef]

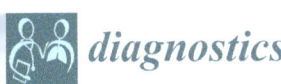

Article

Using High-Resolution Ultrasound to Assess Post-Facial Paralysis Synkinesis—Machine Settings and Technical Aspects for Facial Surgeons

Andreas Kehrer [1,*], Marc Ruewe [1], Natascha Platz Batista da Silva [2], Daniel Lonic [1], Paul Immanuel Heidekrueger [1], Samuel Knoedler [3], Ernst Michael Jung [2], Lukas Prantl [1] and Leonard Knoedler [1]

1. Department of Plastic, Hand and Reconstructive Surgery, University Hospital Regensburg, 93053 Regensburg, Germany; marc.ruewe@ukr.de (M.R.); lonic@mclinic.de (D.L.); post@dr.heidekrueger.de (P.I.H.); lukas.prantl@ukr.de (L.P.); leonard.knoedler@stud.uni-regensburg.de (L.K.)
2. Department of Radiology, University Hospital Regensburg, 93053 Regensburg, Germany; natascha.platz-batista-da-silva@ukr.de (N.P.B.d.S.); ernst-michael.jung@ukr.de (E.M.J.)
3. Department of Plastic Surgery and Hand Surgery, Klinikum Rechts der Isar, Technical University of Munich, 81675 Munich, Germany; samuel.knoedler@tum.de
* Correspondence: andreaskehrer@gmx.de; Tel.: +49-941-944-6763

Abstract: Background: Synkinesis of the facial musculature is a detrimental sequalae in post-paralytic facial palsy (PPFP) patients. Detailed knowledge on the technical requirements and device properties in a high-resolution ultrasound (HRUS) examination is mandatory for a reliable facial muscle assessment in PPFP patients. We therefore aimed to outline the key steps in a HRUS examination and extract an optimized workflow schema. Methods: From December 2020 to April 2021, 20 patients with unilateral synkinesis underwent HRUS. All HRUS examinations were performed by the first author using US devices with linear multifrequency transducers of 4–18 MHz, including a LOGIQ E9 and a LOGIQ S7 XDclear (GE Healthcare; Milwaukee, WI, USA), as well as Philips Affinity 50G (Philips Health Systems; Eindhoven, the Netherlands). Results: Higher-frequency and multifrequency linear probes ≥ 15 MHz provided superior imaging qualities. The selection of the preset program Small Parts, Breast or Thyroid was linked with a more detailed contrast of the imaging morphology of facial tissue layers. Frequency (Frq) = 15 MHz, Gain (Gn) = 25–35 db, Depth (D) = 1–1.5 cm, and Focus (F) = 0.5 cm enhanced the image quality and assessability. Conclusions: An optimized HRUS examination protocol for quantitative and qualitative facial muscle assessments was proposed.

Keywords: Depressor Anguli Oris; zygomaticus major; high-resolution ultrasound; facial reanimation; synkinesis; natural smile; facial surgery; facial symmetry; facial palsy; smile restoration

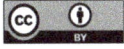

1. Introduction

Facial palsy (FP) patients present with a wide array of muscular, connective, and soft tissue pathologies correlated with different severity levels and comorbidities [1–6]. Dysfunctional facial mimic movements constitute a hallmark of FP sequalae and can tremendously impair a patient's psychological health, social interaction, and overall quality of life [7–10]. The orchestration of the facial musculature to adequately express a plethora of emotional states is complex and finely balanced [11–13]. Research works have shed light on this muscular network in the specific setting of FP [14–17]. The key muscles for facial symmetry and physiological smile movement have been carved out in micro- and macroanatomical studies [18–21]. As a protagonist muscle in the perioral region, the Depressor Anguli Oris (DAO) muscle displays a linear origin from the mental tubercle and is inserted on average into the modiolus 10 mm lateral and 10 mm caudal to the oral commissure. Under its muscle tissue, the mental nerve emerges from the mental foramen and connects to the buccal branch (BB) and marginal mandibular branch (MMB) of the facial nerve [21–23]. While the BB usually pierces the middle-third of the lateral border of the DAO, the MMB passes the DAO through the lower-third of the lateral border. In PPFP, this phenomenon of DAO dual innervation may be the underlying cause of its hypertonicity in contrast to the weakened Depressor Labii Inferioris (DLI) muscle, which is singly innervated by the MMB [23,24]. Of note, the MMB is commonly represented by one or two branches [25]. The microanatomy of the MMB has been studied by our group previously, demonstrating its axonal load, fascicle structure, and diameter [18,26]. With its function of lowering the corner of the mouth, the DAO is crucial for expressing sorrow and anger, for example [27]. Further, the Zygomaticus Major (ZM) is a cornerstone in the human smile movement [28,29]. The ZM originates at the inferolateral part of the malar eminence in the subzygomatic fossa and runs to the modiolar area [30,31]. Throughout its anatomical course, its appearance shifts from a cylindric shape to a bifid architecture at its insertion locus in 30% of cases [32,33]. This anatomical feature may be the underlying reason for the formation of cheek dimples [28]. The ZM is typically supplied by the facial artery, which pierces its muscular bands in 40% of cases [34]. Raising the corner of the mouth, it is involved in the expression of joy and happiness and thus can be considered, to some extent, a functional opponent to the DAO [28].

The DAO muscle has aroused interest in FP therapy, as its unbalanced and unvoluntary contraction causes a distinctive deformity and divergence between the emotional state and facial expression [27,35–37]. DAO dysfunction is indirectly aggravated in FP patients presenting with weakened ZM, since the antagonizing and balancing pull of the ZM is reduced [38,39]. In synkinetic FP patients, these pathognomonic characteristics are particularly prominent [40].

To provide FP patients with adequate and individualized therapy, the diagnostic procedure and preoperative planning tools should be reliable, reproduceable, easy-to-use, widely available, and cost-effective.

The heterogeneous etiology and pathology of FP have counteracted efforts towards general recommendations in FP therapy and diagnostics. For example, the FP therapy guidelines of different associations include varying recommendations regarding the routine diagnostic imaging in new onset FP cases while generally outlining the value of a thorough clinical examination in combination with advanced diagnostic steps [41,42]. However, there is a mounting body of evidence suggesting the beneficial use of high-resolution ultrasound (HRUS) in conjunction with a thorough clinical examination in FP patients, as well as corroborating the overall advancement in visualization quality of a HRUS examination [43–47]. Yet, a step-by-step HRUS examination routine for facial muscle assessment remains to be developed.

While fulfilling the diverse requirements for clinically applicable diagnostic features, the HRUS examination technique is easy to learn for facial surgeons and may enlarge the diagnostic arsenal. A recent scientific work done by Volk et al. underscored the relevance of device settings for small parts imaging [48,49]. Kehrer et al. proposed defined step-by-step algorithms for US machine settings and the visualization and characterization of microvessels [50,51].

The present study aimed to evaluate the technical requirements and different HRUS device properties for facial muscle imaging in PPFP patients showing synkinesis. It was therefore planned to provide a starting guide for facial surgeons less experienced in or even novice at US technology. Based on the results, an optimized HRUS sequence for facial muscle assessment, including the identification of morphologic landmarks and muscular diameter measurement, is proposed. Further, the dynamic evaluation of muscular movement in the DAO region is depicted.

2. Materials and Methods

From December 2020 to April 2021, a prospective data acquisition and analysis of US data was conducted on 20 patients seen at the Department of Plastic, Hand, and

Reconstructive Surgery at the University Hospital Regensburg, Germany. The inclusion criteria comprised patients featuring a pathologic Sunnybrook Facial Grading System score regarding synkinesis [52]. All HRUS examinations were performed by the first author using US devices with linear multifrequency transducers of 4–18 MHz, including a LOGIQ E9 and a LOGIQ S7 XDclear (GE Healthcare; Milwaukee, WI, USA), as well as Philips Affinity 50G (Philips Health Systems; Eindhoven, the Netherlands). The last author supervised each examination over the entire course and ensured proper prospective data collection. A single-examiner HRUS examination was conducted, providing a consistent and identical workflow in the context of US representing a highly operator-dependent technology [53]. Institutional board review and informed consent were obtained prior to the study.

2.1. High-Resolution Brightness (B)-Mode Examination

B-mode is a basic 2D mode and should lay the groundwork for every US examination. Echo-producing interfaces are scanned by the matrix or linear arrays of transducers in the ultrasound probe. The position of the echo is determined by the time window between the acoustical pulse and its echo, as well as the angular positioning of the transducer. The individual pixel brightness is modulated by the amplitude of the returning US signal. Of note, the typical real-time grayscale picture is formed by the echoes of various acoustic impedances from different tissue layers.

2.2. Practical Methodology and Identification of Fundamental Knobology

Useful knobs, switches, and buttons for the assessment of the facial muscle morphology and characteristics in post-facial paralysis synkinesis should be identified and outlined.

2.3. Standardized Workflow Protocol

Vital elements of the US exam were disaggregated into key steps for safe facial muscle identification and characterization. A standardized protocol for the US exams was applied.

For the purpose of the present study, the focus was set on the visualization of the DAO muscle morphology, measuring the muscular diameter, and assessing the dynamic behavior in a real-time US examination. The device settings providing specific values for the Frequency (Frq), Gain (Gn), Depth (D), and Focus (F) should be analyzed for an optimized imaging of the facial muscle morphology.

3. Results

3.1. Technical Requirements

The implementation of a new generation high-resolution US device is recommended. The upcoming generation of US devices accumulates various advancements, including refined reporting features and security measures and improved tissue characterization, as well as novel super-resolution techniques [54]. To this end, US machines should be equipped with high-performance computer chips, typically integrated in the larger pushable-type machines rather than in the portable-type handheld devices.

3.2. Practical Methodology

Many ultrasound devices share strong similarities of steering panels. The knobology of a standard ultrasound device panel is outlined for the mimetic muscle examiner in Figure 1. Adapted to the specific needs of facial surgeons, useful knobs, switches, and buttons to adjust the parameters are subcategorized into different functional groups in Table 1.

3.3. Transducer Selection, Preset Programs, and Device Properties

In this study, higher frequency and multifrequency linear probes ≥ 15 MHz were helpful adjustments for detecting facial muscles, as well as providing enhanced imaging qualities. Selection of the preset program Small Parts, Breast or Thyroid was linked with a more detailed contrast of the imaging morphology of facial tissue layers in B-mode.

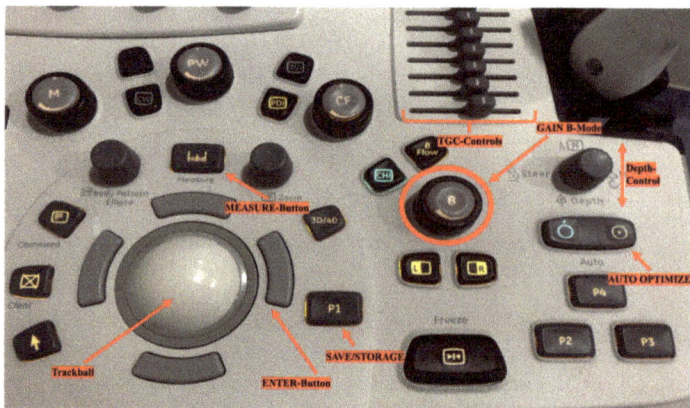

Figure 1. Knobology of a standard ultrasound (US) device. Useful buttons for simplified US usage are marked in red. Time gain controls (TCG) may be all set in the middle position. The depth is varied by the upper and lower lever actions (far right, up). The "Auto Optimize" button harmonizes the image quality. P1 can be programmed to save/store images (in freeze) or cine loops (in a nonfrozen visualization).

3.4. Practical Sequence, Structured Approach, and Standardized Workflow Protocol

In B-mode, the morphology of the skin, subcutaneous, fascia (SMAS), and muscle tissue are depicted (Figure 2). The use of one focus/foci helped to improve the image quality in the targeted area. B-mode images can be optimized with regards to the focus and depth level settings, as well as the preset selection for optimal tissue layer identification. Assessment of the facial tissues is conducted with a superficial high-resolution scan in B-Mode. The centimeter bar located on the right side of the screen helped in the identification and distinction of tissue layers. The dermis and muscle fascia are hyperechoic (bright). In between, fatty components of the subcutaneous and SMAS tissue appear less echoic (darker) in comparison to the dermis.

Table 1. Functional classification of ultrasound (US) knobology. Group A comprises on-screen options and knobs to store patient data, probe the selection, and classify the ultrasound findings for saved images. Group B includes knobs, switches, and buttons that help to adjust the Contrast, Frequency, Focus, Depth, and other settings. Group C summarizes the functions to quantify distances using a measuring tool.

Knobology for Facial Muscle Assessment with Ultrasound (US)			
Group A	Pre-exam buttons	On Display	Patient data button, Probe selection button (usually different linear and convex probes selectable), On-screen buttons for different program presets
	Knobs to classify ultrasound findings for saved pictures		Text editing button
			Body pattern ellipse

Table 1. *Cont.*

	Knobology for Facial Muscle Assessment with Ultrasound (US)	
Group B	Adjusting Contrast, Frequency, and Focus	Time Gain Control (TGC) switches
		Gain of B-Mode picture
		Automated Setting Optimization
		Focus, Frequency
	Basic knobs, switches, and buttons	Trackball and Enter-Button
		Depth
		Freeze
		Save Button (fixed images and cine loops, individually programmable)

Table 1. *Cont.*

Knobology for Facial Muscle Assessment with Ultrasound (US)			
Group C	Buttons for measurements	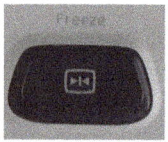	Freeze
		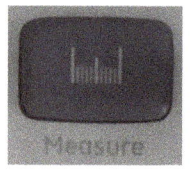	Distance Measurement
		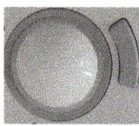	Trackball, Enter

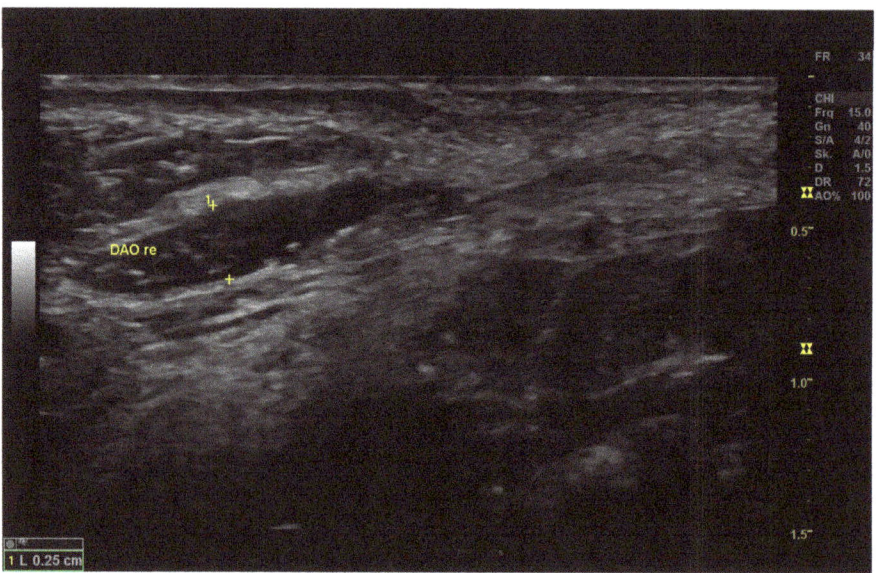

Figure 2. Morphology of the Depressor Anguli Oris (DAO) in the high-resolution brightness (B)-mode examination. Using the preset program Small Parts and the B-mode, the DAO is depicted on the patient's right facial side. Frq = Frequency [Hz].

Key elements of the US examination for efficient and reliable facial muscle identification are summarized in Figure 3. Note that the B-mode should be adjusted and optimized individually for each patient, with an identical sequence for efficiency.

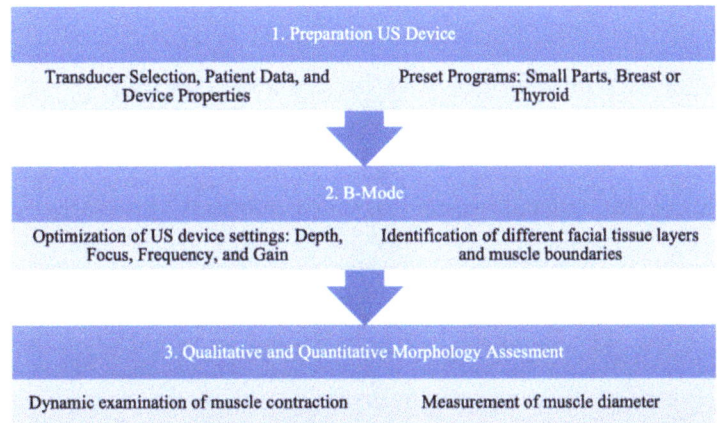

Figure 3. Standardized ultrasound (US) protocol for an effective facial muscle examination. First, the US device is to be prepared for the following examination by selecting an appropriate transducer and preset program. Next step, the brightness (B)-mode can be used to determine different facial tissue layers. Finally, the qualitative and quantitative assessments of muscular morphological features is performed by measuring the cross-sectional muscular diameter and evaluating the muscle functionality in motion.

3.5. Specific Device Settings

Table 2 provides data of specific US settings for optimized facial muscle assessment.

Table 2. High-resolution ultrasound (HRUS) settings to examine the functionality and morphology of facial muscles. The following settings allow for the precise assessment of morphological and functional features during a facial muscle examination.

Facial Muscle Morphology in Ultrasound (US) Examination	
B-mode (B)	
Probe selection	linear (optimal 15–18 MHz)
Frequency (Frq)	15 MHz
Gain (Gn)	25–35 db
Depth (D)	1–1.5 cm
Focus (F)	0.5 cm

3.6. Cross-Sectional Diameter of Facial Muscles

To assess and objectify post-FP synkinesis, facial muscle cross-sectional diameters can be measured at their midpoint in repose and during maximal contraction. Adjusting the depth and magnification helped to increase the precision.

3.7. Practical Sequence and Structured Approach

A structured step-by-step approach decisively shortened the examination times. An examination of related muscles in both facial halves helped to distinguish pathological patterns. Thus, a useful sequence may comprise the following steps:

i. Start with using the B-Mode settings and identify the different tissue layers, such as the skin, subcutaneous, fascia (SMAS), and muscle tissue.
ii. Apply the freeze function and measure the diameter of the facial muscles at their midpoint. Do not forget to store the pictures before unfreezing.
iii. For a dynamic examination, ask the patient to repetitively perform a broad smile and save the cine loops.

The assessment of dynamic muscle behavior in a real-time US examination using the cine loop function is demonstrated in Video S1.

4. Discussion

Facial muscle dysfunction impairs the patient's quality of life on multiple levels, affecting the oral functionality and mimetic communication [1,3,55]. Thus, effective, reproduceable, and unbiased diagnostic procedures lay the groundwork for introducing targeted therapy concepts in an early post-onset stage. Undoubtedly, the clinical inspection of facial muscles represents a powerful tool in the hands of experienced examiners; yet, it remains subjective. This underscores the necessity to objectify facial muscle malfunction in repose and dynamic movement. HRUS combines wide availability, objective measurements, efficient work- and time flows, noninvasiveness, and cost-effectiveness [56]. Recent advancements in HRUS technology have opened this field for facial surgeons and any specialty involved in the treatment of PPFP cases [50,51,57,58]. To successfully perform an US examination, the facial surgeon and examiner only need a little, yet structured, training, which may be acquired through basic ultrasound courses focusing on the vascular system.

The present work described further how to precisely set ultrasound devices to make them applicable for assessing PPFP and its typical symptoms. It is supposed to address facial surgeons and other disciplines interested in familiarizing themselves with HRUS. Thus, a structured workflow algorithm is proposed to depict and objectify structural (morphological), static, and dynamic facial muscle changes in PPFP. Therefore, to further subdivide the ultrasound technology eligible for facial muscle evaluation, a step-by-step guide providing different steps was now defined in this study. This new structured approach may aid less experienced examiners or even novices in HRUS to gain a clearer view into US technology. Concrete setting values for the Frequency (Frq), Gain (Gn), Focus (F), and Depth (D) for a targeted HRUS examination are provided.

To this end, we used US devices favoring a 15–18-MHz transducer, which is comparable to most contemporary pushable US machine available in almost any larger hospital.

We also underscore that the exact machine settings for facial muscle imaging are indispensable for an efficacious execution. Further, a structured approach using a standardized US mode sequence enhanced the work speed and efficiency in the present study. The authors had previously spent circa 30 min performing HRUS on the face. By applying the proposed sequenced protocol, the examination times could be relevantly reduced to 15–20 min. In addition, US allowed for the efficient measurement of a cross-sectional facial muscle diameter. Visualization of the dynamic facial muscle behavior in PPFP and other types of FP may enhance the examiner's understanding of the pathological features of muscle morphology. Thus, US may represent a helpful tool in FP diagnostics and may affect the selection of different treatments, such as surgical concepts in the future. Of note, the surgical concepts can be classified into static and dynamic procedures [59,60]. In hyperactive DAO and ZM, dynamic techniques, such as DAO myectomy, selective neurectomy, and Botulinum Toxin A, are valuable therapy options [61]. Rozen et al. showed that the patient achieved significantly enhanced smile excursion following DAO myectomy [62]. DAO muscle transfer as first described by Klebuc et al. may provide symmetrical enhancement in repose and in motion [63–65]. The concept reroutes the DAO's antagonizing downward pull at the modiolus in a smile. This may facilitate the oblique and superior muscle contractility of smile muscles, such as the ZM. Further, the rerouted DAO may enhance the muscular functions of the DLI, which is often found to be dysfunctional in synkinetic patients.

Future studies involving HRUS could investigate facial muscles changes occurring postoperatively, as well as following conservative management. US applying 3D technology or a volumetric assessment may reveal intramuscular changes associated with different (non-)surgical procedures [66]. Further studies are needed to determine how US morphologic and functional findings, such as (facial) muscle size and dynamic muscular behavior, correlate with clinical conditions like muscular hypertonicity. It is the wish of the authors of this paper that, based on the publication of adequate device settings, further US studies are stimulated in the future that contribute to a better understanding of the underlying muscular changes in PPFP.

Limitations

The results of this study ought to be interpreted in light of the following limitations: The set-up of the US algorithm is based on observational findings in 20 patients with PPFP. While the findings need to be corroborated in larger-scale studies, the sample comprises the most commonly encountered clinical scenarios of PPFP cases. Further, the elucidating research work in this field featured comparable sample sizes [62].

5. Conclusions

The proposed US device settings for facial muscle examination may facilitate the facial surgeon's workflow and result in an enhanced image quality. The structured working protocol may especially help US beginners in conducting more insightful examinations in PFPS patients.

Supplementary Materials: The following supporting information can be downloaded at https://www.mdpi.com/article/10.3390/diagnostics12071650/s1: Video S1. Case example for contrary contraction patterns of nonaffected and synkinetic Depressor Anguli Oris muscles (DAO). The video sequence demonstrates a dynamic HRUS examination comparing DAO morphology in both facial halves while the patient performs a closed-lip smile. On the nonaffected side, the DAO is being stretched while smiling. On the synkinetic side, however, the muscle bulk and cross-sectional diameter of the DAO increase during the smile movement.

Author Contributions: Conceptualization, A.K. and L.K.; methodology, A.K., M.R. and L.K.; software, N.P.B.d.S. and E.M.J.; validation, A.K., M.R., D.L. and P.I.H.; formal analysis, A.K., N.P.B.d.S. and L.K.; investigation, A.K., M.R. and L.K.; resources, A.K., N.P.B.d.S. and E.M.J.; data curation, A.K., S.K. and L.K.; writing—original draft preparation, A.K. and L.K.; writing—review and editing, M.R., N.P.B.d.S., D.L., P.I.H. and L.P.; visualization, M.R., N.P.B.d.S. and P.I.H.; supervision, E.M.J. and L.P.; and project administration, A.K. and L.P. All authors have read and agreed to the published version of the manuscript.

Funding: This research received no external funding.

Institutional Review Board Statement: The study was conducted in accordance with the Declaration of Helsinki and approved by the Institutional Review Board of University of Regensburg (18-1133-101; Date of approval: 19 December 2018).

Informed Consent Statement: Informed consent was obtained from all subjects involved in the study. Written informed consent was obtained from the patients to publish this paper.

Data Availability Statement: Not applicable.

Conflicts of Interest: The authors declare no conflict of interest.

References

1. Zhang, W.; Xu, L.; Luo, T.; Wu, F.; Zhao, B.; Li, X. The etiology of Bell's palsy: A review. *J. Neurol.* **2020**, *267*, 1896–1905. [CrossRef] [PubMed]
2. Lassaletta, L.; Morales-Puebla, J.M.; Altuna, X.; Arbizu, Á.; Arístegui, M.; Batuecas, Á.; Cenjor, C.; Espinosa-Sánchez, J.M.; García-Iza, L.; García-Raya, P.; et al. Facial paralysis: Clinical practice guideline of the Spanish Society of Otolaryngology. *Acta Otorrinolaringol. (Engl. Ed.)* **2020**, *71*, 99–118. [CrossRef]
3. Shokri, T.; Azizzadeh, B.; Ducic, Y. Modern Management of Facial Nerve Disorders. *Semin. Plast. Surg.* **2020**, *34*, 277–285. [CrossRef] [PubMed]
4. Heckmann, J.G.; Urban, P.P.; Pitz, S.; Guntinas-Lichius, O. The Diagnosis and Treatment of Idiopathic Facial Paresis (Bell's Palsy). *Dtsch. Arztebl. Int.* **2019**, *116*, 692–702. [CrossRef]
5. Bylund, N.; Jensson, D.; Enghag, S.; Berg, T.; Marsk, E.; Hultcrantz, M.; Hadziosmanovic, N.; Rodriguez-Lorenzo, A.; Jonsson, L. Synkinesis in Bell's palsy in a randomised controlled trial. *Clin. Otolaryngol.* **2017**, *42*, 673–680. [CrossRef]
6. Park, J.M.; Kim, M.G.; Jung, J.; Kim, S.S.; Jung, A.R.; Kim, S.H.; Yeo, S.G. Effect of Age and Severity of Facial Palsy on Taste Thresholds in Bell's Palsy Patients. *J. Audiol. Otol.* **2017**, *21*, 16–21. [CrossRef]

7. Miller, M.Q.; Hadlock, T.A. Beyond Botox: Contemporary Management of Nonflaccid Facial Palsy. *Facial Plast. Surg. Aesthet. Med.* **2020**, *22*, 65–70. [CrossRef]
8. Parsa, K.M.; Hancock, M.; Nguy, P.L.; Donalek, H.M.; Wang, H.; Barth, J.; Reilly, M.J. Association of Facial Paralysis with Perceptions of Personality and Physical Traits. *JAMA Netw. Open* **2020**, *3*, e205495. [CrossRef]
9. Li, M.K.; Niles, N.; Gore, S.; Ebrahimi, A.; McGuinness, J.; Clark, J.R. Social perception of morbidity in facial nerve paralysis. *Head Neck* **2016**, *38*, 1158–1163. [CrossRef]
10. Fujiwara, K.; Furuta, Y.; Aoki, W.; Nakamaru, Y.; Morita, S.; Hoshino, K.; Fukuda, A.; Homma, A. Make-Up Therapy for Patients with Facial Nerve Palsy. *Ann. Otol. Rhinol. Laryngol.* **2019**, *128*, 721–727. [CrossRef]
11. Schumann, N.P.; Bongers, K.; Scholle, H.C.; Guntinas-Lichius, O. Atlas of voluntary facial muscle activation: Visualization of surface electromyographic activities of facial muscles during mimic exercises. *PLoS ONE* **2021**, *16*, e0254932. [CrossRef] [PubMed]
12. Freilinger, G.; Gruber, H.; Happak, W.; Pechmann, U. Surgical anatomy of the mimic muscle system and the facial nerve: Importance for reconstructive and aesthetic surgery. *Plast. Reconstr. Surg.* **1987**, *80*, 686–690. [CrossRef] [PubMed]
13. Diogo, R.; Wood, B.A.; Aziz, M.A.; Burrows, A. On the origin, homologies and evolution of primate facial muscles, with a particular focus on hominoids and a suggested unifying nomenclature for the facial muscles of the Mammalia. *J. Anat.* **2009**, *215*, 300–319. [CrossRef] [PubMed]
14. Wenceslau, L.G.; Sassi, F.C.; Magnani, D.M.; Andrade, C.R. Peripheral facial palsy: Muscle activity in different onset times. *Codas* **2016**, *28*, 3–9. [CrossRef] [PubMed]
15. Volk, G.F.; Pohlmann, M.; Sauer, M.; Finkensieper, M.; Guntinas-Lichius, O. Quantitative ultrasonography of facial muscles in patients with chronic facial palsy. *Muscle Nerve* **2014**, *50*, 358–365. [CrossRef]
16. Baba, S.; Kondo, K.; Yamasoba, T. Electrophysiological Evaluation of the Facial Muscles in Congenital Unilateral Lower Lip Palsy. *Otol. Neurotol.* **2018**, *39*, 106–110. [CrossRef]
17. Sauer, M.; Guntinas-Lichius, O.; Volk, G.F. Ultrasound echomyography of facial muscles in diagnosis and follow-up of facial palsy in children. *Eur. J. Paediatr. Neurol.* **2016**, *20*, 666–670. [CrossRef]
18. Mandlik, V.; Ruewe, M.; Engelmann, S.; Geis, S.; Taeger, C.; Kehrer, M.; Tamm, E.R.; Bleys, R.; Prantl, L.; Kehrer, A. Significance of the Marginal Mandibular Branch in Relation to Facial Palsy Reconstruction: Assessment of Microanatomy and Macroanatomy Including Axonal Load in 96 Facial Halves. *Ann. Plast. Surg.* **2019**, *83*, e43–e49. [CrossRef]
19. Ruewe, M.; Engelmann, S.; Huang, C.W.; Klein, S.M.; Anker, A.M.; Lamby, P.; Bleys, R.; Tamm, E.R.; Prantl, L.; Kehrer, A. Microanatomy of the Frontal Branch of the Facial Nerve: The Role of Nerve Caliber and Axonal Capacity. *Plast. Reconstr. Surg.* **2021**, *148*, 1357–1365. [CrossRef]
20. Cotofana, S.; Freytag, D.L.; Frank, K.; Sattler, S.; Landau, M.; Pavicic, T.; Fabi, S.; Lachman, N.; Hernandez, C.A.; Green, J.B. The Bidirectional Movement of the Frontalis Muscle: Introducing the Line of Convergence and Its Potential Clinical Relevance. *Plast. Reconstr. Surg.* **2020**, *145*, 1155–1162. [CrossRef]
21. De Bonnecaze, G.; Vergez, S.; Chaput, B.; Vairel, B.; Serrano, E.; Chantalat, E.; Chaynes, P. Variability in facial-muscle innervation: A comparative study based on electrostimulation and anatomical dissection. *Clin. Anat.* **2019**, *32*, 169–175. [CrossRef]
22. Uygur, S.; Konofaos, P. Topographic and Neural Anatomy of the Depressor Anguli Oris Muscle and Implications for Treatment of Synkinetic Facial Paralysis. *Plast. Reconstr. Surg.* **2022**, *149*, 146e–147e. [CrossRef] [PubMed]
23. Krag, A.E.; Dumestre, D.; Hembd, A.; Glick, S.; Mohanty, A.J.; Rozen, S.M. Topographic and Neural Anatomy of the Depressor Anguli Oris Muscle and Implications for Treatment of Synkinetic Facial Paralysis. *Plast. Reconstr. Surg.* **2021**, *147*, 268e–278e. [CrossRef] [PubMed]
24. Hur, M.S.; Hu, K.S.; Cho, J.Y.; Kwak, H.H.; Song, W.C.; Koh, K.S.; Lorente, M.; Kim, H.J. Topography and location of the depressor anguli oris muscle with a reference to the mental foramen. *Surg. Radiol. Anat.* **2008**, *30*, 403–407. [CrossRef] [PubMed]
25. Marcuzzo, A.V.; Šuran-Brunelli, A.N.; Dal Cin, E.; Rigo, S.; Piccinato, A.; Boscolo Nata, F.; Tofanelli, M.; Boscolo-Rizzo, P.; Grill, V.; Di Lenarda, R.; et al. Surgical Anatomy of the Marginal Mandibular Nerve: A Systematic Review and Meta-Analysis. *Clin. Anat.* **2020**, *33*, 739–750. [CrossRef]
26. Engelmann, S.; Ruewe, M.; Geis, S.; Taeger, C.D.; Kehrer, M.; Tamm, E.R.; Bleys, R.L.A.W.; Zeman, F.; Prantl, L.; Kehrer, A. Rapid and Precise Semi-Automatic Axon Quantification in Human Peripheral Nerves. *Sci. Rep.* **2020**, *10*, 1935. [CrossRef] [PubMed]
27. Jowett, N.; Malka, R.; Hadlock, T.A. Effect of Weakening of Ipsilateral Depressor Anguli Oris on Smile Symmetry in Postparalysis Facial Palsy. *JAMA Facial Plast. Surg.* **2017**, *19*, 29–33. [CrossRef]
28. Pessa, J.E.; Zadoo, V.P.; Garza, P.A.; Adrian, E.K., Jr.; Dewitt, A.I.; Garza, J.R. Double or bifid zygomaticus major muscle: Anatomy, incidence, and clinical correlation. *Clin. Anat.* **1998**, *11*, 310–313. [CrossRef]
29. Kehrer, A.; Engelmann, S.; Bauer, R.; Taeger, C.; Grechenig, S.; Kehrer, M.; Prantl, L.; Tamm, E.; Bleys, R.; Mandlik, V. The nerve supply of zygomaticus major: Variability and distinguishing zygomatic from buccal facial nerve branches. *Clin. Anat.* **2018**, *31*, 560–565. [CrossRef]
30. Miller, P.J.; Smith, S.; Shah, A. The subzygomatic fossa: A practical landmark in identifying the zygomaticus major muscle. *Arch. Facial Plast. Surg.* **2007**, *9*, 271–274. [CrossRef]
31. Wong, C.H.; Mendelson, B. Facial soft-tissue spaces and retaining ligaments of the midcheek: Defining the premaxillary space. *Plast. Reconstr. Surg.* **2013**, *132*, 49–56. [CrossRef] [PubMed]

32. Shim, K.S.; Hu, K.S.; Kwak, H.H.; Youn, K.H.; Koh, K.S.; Fontaine, C.; Kim, H.J. An anatomical study of the insertion of the zygomaticus major muscle in humans focused on the muscle arrangement at the corner of the mouth. *Plast. Reconstr. Surg.* **2008**, *121*, 466–473. [CrossRef] [PubMed]
33. Phan, K.; Onggo, J. Prevalence of Bifid Zygomaticus Major Muscle. *J. Craniofac. Surg.* **2019**, *30*, 758–760. [CrossRef] [PubMed]
34. Kwak, H.H.; Hu, K.S.; Youn, K.H.; Jin, G.C.; Shim, K.S.; Fontaine, C.; Kim, H.J. Topographic relationship between the muscle bands of the zygomaticus major muscle and the facial artery. *Surg. Radiol. Anat.* **2006**, *28*, 477–480. [CrossRef] [PubMed]
35. Liu, M.T.; Iglesias, R.A.; Sekhon, S.S.; Li, Y.; Larson, K.; Totonchi, A.; Guyuron, B. Factors contributing to facial asymmetry in identical twins. *Plast. Reconstr. Surg.* **2014**, *134*, 638–646. [CrossRef]
36. Lee, H.J.; Kim, J.S.; Youn, K.H.; Lee, J.; Kim, H.J. Ultrasound-Guided Botulinum Neurotoxin Type A Injection for Correcting Asymmetrical Smiles. *Aesthet. Surg. J.* **2018**, *38*, NP130–NP134. [CrossRef]
37. Terzis, J.K.; Kalantarian, B. Microsurgical strategies in 74 patients for restoration of dynamic depressor muscle mechanism: A neglected target in facial reanimation. *Plast. Reconstr. Surg.* **2000**, *105*, 1917–1931. [CrossRef]
38. Gray, H. The muscles and fasciae. In *Anatomy, Descriptive and Surgical*; Pick, T.P., Howden, R., Eds.; Pennsylvania State University: State College, PA, USA, 1974; pp. 306–315.
39. de Maio, M.; Rzany, B. *Botulinum Toxin in Aesthetic Medicine*; Springer: Berlin/Heidelberg, Germany, 2007.
40. Leader, B.; Azizzadeh, B. Synkinetic Unilateral Lower Lip Palsy: Diagnosis and Technical Considerations for Facial Reanimation. *Facial Plast. Surg. Aesthet. Med.* **2021**, *23*, 309–311. [CrossRef]
41. Baugh, R.F.; Basura, G.J.; Ishii, L.E.; Schwartz, S.R.; Drumheller, C.M.; Burkholder, R.; Deckard, N.A.; Dawson, C.; Driscoll, C.; Gillespie, M.B.; et al. Clinical practice guideline: Bell's Palsy executive summary. *Otolaryngol. Head Neck Surg.* **2013**, *149*, 656–663. [CrossRef]
42. de Almeida, J.R.; Guyatt, G.H.; Sud, S.; Dorion, J.; Hill, M.D.; Kolber, M.R.; Lea, J.; Reg, S.L.; Somogyi, B.K.; Westerberg, B.D.; et al. Management of Bell palsy: Clinical practice guideline. *Cmaj* **2014**, *186*, 917–922. [CrossRef]
43. Li, S.; Guo, R.J.; Liang, X.N.; Wu, Y.; Cao, W.; Zhang, Z.P.; Zhao, W.; Liang, H.D. High-frequency ultrasound as an adjunct to neural electrophysiology: Evaluation and prognosis of Bell's palsy. *Exp. Ther. Med.* **2016**, *11*, 77–82. [CrossRef] [PubMed]
44. Baek, S.-H.; Kim, Y.H.; Kwon, Y.-J.; Sung, J.H.; Son, M.H.; Lee, J.H.; Kim, B.-J. The Utility of Facial Nerve Ultrasonography in Bell's Palsy. *Otolaryngol. Head Neck Surg.* **2019**, *162*, 186–192. [CrossRef] [PubMed]
45. Zhu, J.; Li, X.; Han, Y.; Cao, Y.; Guan, L.; Geng, X. High frequency ultrasonography of the facial nerve: Another effective method to observe the course of idiopathic facial nerve paralysis. *Environ. Dis.* **2020**, *5*, 100–106. [CrossRef]
46. Tashiro, K.; Yamashita, S.; Araki, J.; Narushima, M.; Iida, T.; Koshima, I. Preoperative color Doppler ultrasonographic examination in the planning of thoracodorsal artery perforator flap with capillary perforators. *J. Plast. Reconstr. Aesthet. Surg.* **2016**, *69*, 346–350. [CrossRef]
47. Su, W.; Lu, L.; Lazzeri, D.; Zhang, Y.X.; Wang, D.; Innocenti, M.; Qian, Y.; Agostini, T.; Levin, L.S.; Messmer, C. Contrast-enhanced ultrasound combined with three-dimensional reconstruction in preoperative perforator flap planning. *Plast. Reconstr. Surg.* **2013**, *131*, 80–93. [CrossRef]
48. Wegscheider, H.; Volk, G.F.; Guntinas-Lichius, O.; Moriggl, B. High-resolution ultrasonography of the normal extratemporal facial nerve. *Eur. Arch. Otorhinolaryngol.* **2018**, *275*, 293–299. [CrossRef]
49. Volk, G.F.; Wystub, N.; Pohlmann, M.; Finkensieper, M.; Chalmers, H.J.; Guntinas-Lichius, O. Quantitative ultrasonography of facial muscles. *Muscle Nerve* **2013**, *47*, 878–883. [CrossRef]
50. Kehrer, A.; Sachanadani, N.S.; da Silva, N.P.B.; Lonic, D.; Heidekrueger, P.; Taeger, C.D.; Klein, S.; Jung, E.M.; Prantl, L.; Hong, J.P. Step-by-step guide to ultrasound-based design of alt flaps by the microsurgeon—Basic and advanced applications and device settings. *J. Plast. Reconstr. Aesthet. Surg.* **2020**, *73*, 1081–1090. [CrossRef]
51. Kehrer, A.; Lonic, D.; Heidekrueger, P.; Bosselmann, T.; Taeger, C.D.; Lamby, P.; Kehrer, M.; Jung, E.M.; Prantl, L.; Platz Batista da Silva, N. Feasibility study of preoperative microvessel evaluation and characterization in perforator flaps using various modes of color-coded duplex sonography (CCDS). *Microsurgery* **2020**, *40*, 750–759. [CrossRef]
52. Ross, B.R.; Fradet, G.; Nedzelski, J.M. Development of a sensitive clinical facial grading system. *Eur. Arch. Otorhinolaryngol.* **1996**, *114*, 380–386. [CrossRef]
53. Stasi, G.; Ruoti, E. A critical evaluation in the delivery of the ultrasound practice: The point of view of the radiologist. *Ital. J. Med.* **2015**, *9*. [CrossRef]
54. Rix, A.; Lederle, W.; Theek, B.; Lammers, T.; Moonen, C.; Schmitz, G.; Kiessling, F. Advanced Ultrasound Technologies for Diagnosis and Therapy. *J. Nucl. Med.* **2018**, *59*, 740–746. [CrossRef] [PubMed]
55. Fuzi, J.; Taylor, A.; Sideris, A.; Meller, C. Does Botulinum Toxin Therapy Improve Quality of Life in Patients with Facial Palsy? *Aesthet. Plast. Surg.* **2020**, *44*, 1811–1819. [CrossRef] [PubMed]
56. Lentz, B.; Fong, T.; Rhyne, R.; Risko, N. A systematic review of the cost-effectiveness of ultrasound in emergency care settings. *Ultrasound. J.* **2021**, *13*, 16. [CrossRef]
57. Kehrer, A.; Mandlik, V.; Taeger, C.; Geis, S.; Prantl, L.; Jung, E.M. Postoperative control of functional muscle flaps for facial palsy reconstruction: Ultrasound guided tissue monitoring using contrast enhanced ultrasound (CEUS) and ultrasound elastography. *Clin. Hemorheol. Microcirc.* **2017**, *67*, 435–444. [CrossRef]

58. Kehrer, A.; Heidekrueger, P.I.; Lonic, D.; Taeger, C.D.; Klein, S.; Lamby, P.; Sachanadani, N.S.; Jung, E.M.; Prantl, L.; Batista da Silva, N.P. High-Resolution Ultrasound-Guided Perforator Mapping and Characterization by the Microsurgeon in Lower Limb Reconstruction. *J. Reconstr. Microsurg.* **2021**, *37*, 75–82. [CrossRef]
59. Bassilios Habre, S.; Googe, B.J.; Depew, J.B.; Wallace, R.D.; Konofaos, P. Depressor Reanimation After Facial Nerve Paralysis. *Ann. Plast. Surg.* **2019**, *82*, 582–590. [CrossRef]
60. Klebuc, M.J.A. Facial reanimation using the masseter-to-facial nerve transfer. *Plast. Reconstr. Surg.* **2011**, *127*, 1909–1915. [CrossRef]
61. Patel, P.N.; Owen, S.R.; Norton, C.P.; Emerson, B.T.; Bronaugh, A.B.; Ries, W.R.; Stephan, S.J. Outcomes of Buccinator Treatment With Botulinum Toxin in Facial Synkinesis. *JAMA Facial Plast. Surg.* **2018**, *20*, 196–201. [CrossRef]
62. Halani, S.H.; Sanchez, C.V.; Hembd, A.S.; Mohanty, A.J.; Reisch, J.; Rozen, S.M. Depressor Anguli Oris Myectomy versus Transfer to Depressor Labii Inferioris for Facial Symmetry in Synkinetic Facial Paralysis. *J. Reconstr. Microsurg.* **2022**, *38*, 328–334. [CrossRef]
63. Rozen, S.; Redett, R.J.; Zuker, R.M.; Snyder-Warwick, A.K. ASPN/ASRM Combined Panel I: Difficult Cases of Facial Paralysis—Opportunities and Innovations. In Proceedings of the American Society for Peripheral Nerve 2020 Annual Meeting, Fort Lauderdale, FL, USA, 12 January 2020.
64. Klebuc, M.J.A. Introduction to depressor anguli oris muscle transfer. In Proceedings of the 2020 American Society for Reconstructive Mircrosurgery Annual Meeting, Fort Lauderdale, FL, USA, 10–14 January 2020.
65. Klebuc, M.J.A.; Labio-mental Synkinetic Dysfunction Weill Cornell School of Medicine, New York City, NY, USA. Personal communication, 2020.
66. Platz Batista da Silva, N.; Engeßer, M.; Hackl, C.; Brunner, S.; Hornung, M.; Schlitt, H.J.; Evert, K.; Stroszczynski, C.; Jung, E.M. Intraoperative Characterization of Pancreatic Tumors Using Contrast-Enhanced Ultrasound and Shear Wave Elastography for Optimization of Surgical Strategies. *J. Ultrasound. Med.* **2021**, *40*, 1613–1625. [CrossRef] [PubMed]

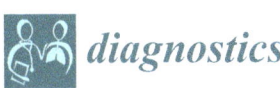

Article

Is There a Difference in Facial Emotion Recognition after Stroke with vs. without Central Facial Paresis?

Anna-Maria Kuttenreich [1,2,3,4,5,*], Harry von Piekartz [6] and Stefan Heim [1,2,7]

1. Department of Psychiatry, Psychotherapy and Psychosomatics, Medical Faculty, RWTH Aachen University, Pauwelsstr. 30, 52074 Aachen, Germany; sheim@ukaachen.de
2. Department of Neurology, Medical Faculty, RWTH Aachen University, Pauwelsstr. 30, 52074 Aachen, Germany
3. Department of Otorhinolaryngology, Jena University Hospital, Am Klinikum 1, 07747 Jena, Germany
4. Facial-Nerve-Center Jena, Jena University Hospital, Am Klinikum 1, 07747 Jena, Germany
5. Center of Rare Diseases Jena, Jena University Hospital, Am Klinikum 1, 07747 Jena, Germany
6. Department of Physical Therapy and Rehabilitation Science, Osnabrück University of Applied Sciences, Albrechtstr. 30, 49076 Osnabrück, Germany; h.von-piekartz@hs-osnabrueck.de
7. Institute of Neuroscience and Medicine (INM-1), Forschungszentrum Jülich, Leo-Brand-Str. 5, 52428 Jülich, Germany
* Correspondence: anna.kuttenreich@rwth-aachen.de; Tel.: +49-3641-9329398

Citation: Kuttenreich, A.-M.; von Piekartz, H.; Heim, S. Is There a Difference in Facial Emotion Recognition after Stroke with vs. without Central Facial Paresis? *Diagnostics* **2022**, *12*, 1721. https://doi.org/10.3390/diagnostics12071721

Academic Editors: Steffen Eisenhardt, Gerd Fabian Volk and Shai Rozen

Received: 12 February 2022
Accepted: 10 July 2022
Published: 15 July 2022

Publisher's Note: MDPI stays neutral with regard to jurisdictional claims in published maps and institutional affiliations.

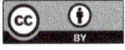

Copyright: © 2022 by the authors. Licensee MDPI, Basel, Switzerland. This article is an open access article distributed under the terms and conditions of the Creative Commons Attribution (CC BY) license (https://creativecommons.org/licenses/by/4.0/).

Abstract: The Facial Feedback Hypothesis (FFH) states that facial emotion recognition is based on the imitation of facial emotional expressions and the processing of physiological feedback. In the light of limited and contradictory evidence, this hypothesis is still being debated. Therefore, in the present study, emotion recognition was tested in patients with central facial paresis after stroke. Performance in facial vs. auditory emotion recognition was assessed in patients with vs. without facial paresis. The accuracy of objective facial emotion recognition was significantly lower in patients with vs. without facial paresis and also in comparison to healthy controls. Moreover, for patients with facial paresis, the accuracy measure for facial emotion recognition was significantly worse than that for auditory emotion recognition. Finally, in patients with facial paresis, the subjective judgements of their own facial emotion recognition abilities differed strongly from their objective performances. This pattern of results demonstrates a specific deficit in facial emotion recognition in central facial paresis and thus provides support for the FFH and points out certain effects of stroke.

Keywords: emotion recognition; facial feedback; central facial paresis; stroke

1. Introduction

Emotion recognition is omnipresent in social interactions [1] and represents an important social competence [2]. Faces provide relevant clues for the recognition of emotions [2,3]. One explanation of the facial recognition of emotions is provided by the Facial Feedback Hypothesis (FFH) [4]. The present study therefore compares stroke patients with vs. without unilateral central facial paresis, i.e., the partial inability to perform facial movements [5], in order to test the FFH prediction of a specific deficit of visual facial emotion recognition in individuals with central facial paresis.

Emotion Processing and the Role of Facial Feedback

Facial emotion expressions are part of nonverbal communication [3] and are regarded as some of the most important nonverbal features in the identification of emotions [6]. Facial expression can be highly variable due to the precise control of the different facial muscles [1] and their voluntary or affective control [7], although the basic emotions framework considers a set of emotions to be highly elementary, unique and independent of culture, time and place [8]. These basic emotions are: anger, disgust, fear, joy, sadness and surprise [9,10]. Each of the basic emotions is characterized by specific patterns of facial muscle activities [8,11]. These congenital, ubiquitous basic emotions [12] are typically used to observe (facial) emotion recognition [13].

The accuracy of emotion recognition varies, depending on the particular emotion presented. Joy is detected significantly more accurately and quickly than all other basic emotions, whereas fear is detected significantly less accurately and more slowly than the other emotions [14]. The basic emotions of surprise and anger, as well as disgust and sadness, are similarly well-identified in terms of accuracy (performance listed in descending order) [14]. Besides differences per emotion, emotion recognition depends on sex and age. Women are faster at facial emotion recognition than men [15]. With increasing age, emotion recognition performance decreases [16]. It has not yet been conclusively clarified whether the processing of emotions is innate [4,17] or whether a concept of emotions must first be learned [18]. A combination is also conceivable, if basic emotions are considered as biologically anchored [12] and innate [17], while all of the other, more complex emotions [8] have to be learned first [12]. The localisation of emotion processing is also a matter of controversy, with evidence for right, left, or left and right hemispheric activation [19]. Dominance of the right hemisphere has been described historically [20], whereas recent evidence has highlighted a combination of different neuronal networks with different lateralization [19].

In emotion processing, the importance of afferent information from the body is emphasised, e.g., facial expression [18]. In this sense, the FFH provides a theoretical account of the process of facial emotion recognition. It postulates that other persons' emotions are recognised by one's own facial information [4]. The decoding requires the imitation of the facial expression of the other person and the corresponding proprioceptive facial feedback [21,22] ('facial reflex' is a synonym for 'facial feedback' [11]). Neal and Chartrand [22] summarised the working steps of the FFH: (1) imitation of the facial expression of the communication partner (discrete, unconscious, fast, automated and specific to the emotion); (2) transmission of afferent information from the face to the brain; and (3) experience and recognition of the emotion [22].

Whereas a person's spontaneous, quick and unobtrusive imitation with their own face is basically unproblematic [23], pathological conditions affecting facial integrity may affect the abilities to initiate or imitate basic emotions' corresponding facial expressions. Such conditions include, for example, facial paresis, a unilateral or bilateral palsy of the facial musculature following a peripheral or central defect [24]. The central form of facial paresis considered in this study typically presents unilaterally, contralateral to the central lesion [25], after stroke [26].

Whether and precisely what role facial feedback plays in emotion recognition has not yet been conclusively clarified. For example, different research results show evidence for and against the FFH in the case of limited facial feedback (due to illness or artificially provoked).

Significant deficits in facial emotion recognition were reported by Konnerth et al. [27] and Storbeck et al. [28] in patients with peripheral facial paresis/paralysis. Konnerth et al. [27] reported that patients achieved lower accuracy values than healthy controls, although the difference was not significant. Storbeck et al. [28] also detected that accuracy in facial emotion recognition did not differ significantly between patients with facial paresis and healthy controls. However, visual emotion recognition was significantly slower compared to the control subjects in both studies [27,28]. More specifically, Korb et al. [29] reported differences depending on the paralysed side of the face, with facial emotion recognition being more affected in patients with left-sided rather than right-sided facial palsy. Such findings might be taken as supportive evidence for the FFH, as persons with intact feedback show faster facial emotion recognition times [22,30–33]. This reduced accuracy of emotion recognition in patients with peripheral facial palsy could be explained by Niedenthal et al. [33], according to whom self-experienced emotions can be recognized earlier than those that are not self-perceived [33]. In contrast, Keillor et al. [34] did not report differences in the accuracy of emotion naming, discrimination or matching tasks in their single case study of a patient with bilateral facial paralysis in Guillain–Barré syndrome, nor did Bogart and Matsumoto [35] report facial emotion recognition deficits in patients with congenital bilateral facial paresis in Moebius syndrome. However, Calder et al. [36] did observe differences in the accuracy of emotion recognition with respect to at least one basic emotion in patients with Moebius syndrome.

A different way of investigating facial feedback in healthy participants is with an injection of botulinum toxin in the facial muscles for temporarily paralysis. Different studies using this method showed changed emotion recognition in terms of accuracy and time [22,32]. The results may point to a direct link between facial feedback and emotion processing [32].

Besides limited facial movements due to experimental induction and peripheral facial palsy, other disorders could also affect (1) facial movements and (2) facial emotion recognition—for instance, central facial palsy after stroke and Parkinson's disease. Stroke occurs suddenly due to disturbed blood flow and oxygen deficiency (ischemic stroke) or bleeding (hemorrhagic stroke) in the brain and leads to individual disabilities [37], whereas Parkinson's disease is a neurodegenerative disorder involving loss of dopamine in the substantia nigra, resulting in typical symptoms of rigor, tremor and bradykinesia [38]. Both central facial palsy after stroke [26,39] and Parkinson's disease [40–42] could result in similar effects, i.e., reduced facial expression and therefore reduced facial feedback. Following the FFH, facial feedback due to facial integrity is needed for facial emotion recognition [23]. Both in stroke [43] and in Parkinson's disease [41], facial emotion recognition could be impaired. However, there is not necessarily a direct correlation between limitations in facial expression and facial emotion recognition, at least in Parkinson's disease [41].

In summary, there is evidence that patients with limited facial feedback and facial mimicry abilities (e.g., in peripheral facial paresis) are potentially affected by limited facial emotion recognition. To date, to the best of our knowledge, patients with peripheral facial palsy have been studied, whereas patients with central facial palsy have been overlooked.

The care of patients with central facial palsy is insufficient and rehabilitation guidelines are required [44]. To improve treatment and establish guidelines, deficits or remaining abilities must be identified first. To this end, we designed a study to find proof of facial emotion recognition abilities in patients with central facial palsy.

Consequently, the aim of the study was to test facial emotion recognition in patients with central facial paresis after stroke in terms of accuracy and time with visually presented, i.e., facial, stimuli presented by healthy subjects. Testing different modalities (facial and auditory) in two patient groups (with or without facial paresis after stroke) allows assessment of whether there is a general deficit in emotion recognition—which is a possibility after stroke [43]—or whether only one particular modality is (more) affected. If there are no deficits in emotion recognition at all, i.e., if the performance is comparable to that of healthy control subjects, it can assume that emotion recognition may be intact. Accordingly, the primary research question was: Can patients with central facial paresis after stroke recognise facial emotions?

2. Materials and Methods

2.1. Participants

Three groups of participants were considered for this study: (1) patients with unilateral central facial paresis after stroke, (2) patients without facial paresis after stroke and (3) healthy subjects. The data for the patient groups (1) and (2) were collected within the study (data are available from the authors on request), whereas the reference values for the healthy subject group (3) were already available [45–47] and served for an additional comparison.

The inclusion and exclusion criteria are summarised in Table 1. The patients were referred by various cooperation partners, hospitals and local practices for speech–language therapy. Recruitment and data collection took place in the period from 22 February until 14 May 2019 in Germany.

Table 1. Inclusion and exclusion criteria.

Inclusion Criteria	Exclusion Criteria
Adult persons ($\geq$18 years) with or without unilateral central facial paresis after stroke (ischemic or hemorrhagic)	Children and adults with peripheral facial paresis
Acute, post-acute or chronic phase of stroke	Other neurological or psychological diseases
For the investigation: - Capacity for approximately 75 min, sitting for approximately 10 min - Ability to choose answer options - Communication skills needed to follow instructions and to answer questionnaires	For the investigation: - Impairment of general status, communication skills and/or ability to answer such that the investigation would not be possible
Normal or corrected visual and hearing ability	
Ability to consent	No ability to consent

A total of 67 patients were recruited. Four of these were drop-out cases (one case: disorientation; one case: suspected bucco–facial apraxia with no possibility of assessing facial paresis; two cases: antidepressant medication with suspected altered emotional regulation). The remaining 63 patients were assigned to the study group (patients with central facial paresis, n = 34) or the control group (patients without facial paresis, n = 29) according to their diagnosis of facial paresis. Sociodemographic data and information on lesions, facial paresis, general mental capacities and aphasia for the study and control groups are given in Tables A1–A3, A5 and A6 (Appendix A).

The study was approved by the local ethics committee (key: EK 271/18) of the Medical Faculty at RWTH Aachen University, and all regulations of the ethics committee were implemented. All experiments were performed in accordance with the relevant guidelines and regulations. All participants signed an informed consent form after receiving detailed information.

2.2. Materials

For both facial emotion recognition and auditory emotion recognition, the same conditions were set, i.e., an item was presented (visually or auditorily) and the patients had ten seconds to respond. There were different options available as answers. The respective software systems recorded accuracy and time. For both modalities, a pre-test with ten items (initially randomized, later presented in the same order) was performed. The pre-test ensured that the task was understood [48] (see, also, Appendix B).

2.2.1. Visual Facial Emotion Recognition

In our study, we opted to use the *Myfacetraining* (MFT) Program (CRAFTA Cranio Facial Therapy Academy, Hamburg, Germany) [47,49], which consists of a standard test for accuracy and time taken for facial emotion recognition [47,49]. Forty-two subjects, each showing a basic emotion with their face, were presented on a screen. The person was first shown in a neutral position before changing to an emotional facial expression (basic emotion). Six additional answer options were displayed on the screen according to the basic emotion [47] (see, also, Appendix B).

2.2.2. Auditory Emotion Recognition

In addition to faces, voices (auditory) are the most important modalities in emotional communication [1]. A sub-portion of the *Montreal Affective Voices (MAVs)* [45] was used for the assessment. These are emotional, non-linguistic, vocal expressions of /a/ (to be compared with *a* as in *apple*, British English). Sixty items for the six basic emotions [45] were used. The *Montreal Affective Voices* were presented with a specially programmed experiment with the software *PsychoPy*, version 3.0.0b9 [50] (see, also, Appendix B).

2.2.3. Subjective Facial Emotion Recognition: Self-Assessment Questionnaires, Emotion Recognition

Coulson et al. [51] asked relatives of patients with facial paresis for their assessments of emotional recognition. Based on this, two standardized questionnaires were designed for the present study which enabled the systematic collection of subjective facial emotion recognition data. The *Self-Assessment Questionnaires Emotion Recognition Accuracy* and *Time* were used to document self-assessment of facial emotion recognition of the six basic emotions (anger, disgust, fear, joy, sadness and surprise) [51]. In order to be able to look at the evaluation in a differentiated way, one questionnaire was developed to assess accuracy and another was developed to assess time taken for facial emotion recognition. The questionnaires assess possible changes between pre-morbid and current abilities per basic emotion. The questions that featured in the questionnaires in each case were as follows: *How well do you recognize the following feelings in other people's faces?* One of three answer options could be selected for each questionnaire. For *Accuracy*, the patient evaluated whether the basic emotion in question was *more difficult, just as well as* or *more easily* recognised than before stroke. For *Time*, the patient indicated whether the basic emotion was detected *slower, as fast as* or *faster* than before stroke. For deteriorations (indicated by the response options *more difficult* or *slower*), a score of -1 was assigned. If the patient did not notice any changes (response options *just as well as* or *just as fast as*), zero points (0) were recorded. For improvements (answer options *easier* or *faster*), the patient achieved a score of $+1$, resulting in a score between -6 and $+6$ per questionnaire.

2.2.4. Sunnybrook Facial Grading System for Diagnosing Facial Paresis

In order to answer the main research question, all patients were examined in a standardised way to identify possible facial paresis. Only this allowed to divide the patients into the study group (participants with central facial paresis) or the control group (participants without central facial paresis). The *Sunnybrook Facial Grading System* [52,53] is used for the standardised assessment for diagnosing facial paresis or paralysis, respectively. This measurement method is explicitly recommended [54]. It is also considered the current standard in the evaluation of facial paresis [55] and has been used in various studies (e.g., [54,56–62]). Ross et al. [52] published the original version of the *Sunnybrook Facial Grading System* in 1996, which was implemented in the present study (German version [53]). For this purpose, a video was made of each patient with an *Apple iPod touch* (camera at right angles, at the individual height of the chewing plane, 150 cm from the patient's chin), in which the patients were asked in a standardised manner to show their face at rest or to perform an arbitrary movement with their face (raise eyebrows, close eyes gently, smile with open mouth, show teeth, pucker lips). The videos were evaluated by a speech–language therapist (see, also, Appendix B).

2.3. Statistical Analysis

Two-factorial ANOVAs with post-hoc *t*-tests were performed with the factors *group* (with vs. without facial paresis) as between-subject factor and *modality* (facial vs. auditory emotion recognition) as within-subject factor. Accuracy and time taken for emotion recognition were considered as dependent variables. In order to compare the empirical data obtained in the present study with normative data for healthy controls (without stroke and without facial paresis) which were already available, a series of *t*-tests were subsequently performed separately both for accuracy and time. To compare facial emotion recognition and auditory emotion recognition in terms of accuracy and time in patients and healthy subjects, *t*-tests were performed for one sample. For the comparison between patients with and without facial paresis, two-factorial ANOVAs and (post-hoc) *t*-tests for independent samples were run. *t*-tests for dependent samples were performed to compare facial emotion recognition and auditory emotion recognition in patients with and without facial paresis. To analyse subjective emotion recognition in terms of accuracy and time, one-sample *t*-tests were conducted. To compare accuracy and time, *t*-tests for dependent samples were performed.

Benjamini–Hochberg correction was applied if more than one *t*-test was conducted.

3. Results

The results for objective (accuracy and time) and subjectively perceived success in emotion recognition are summarised in Figure 1, Figure 2, Figure 3, Figure 4 and Table A4 (Appendix A).

3.1. Accuracy of Facial Emotion Recognition

The results of the ANOVA for accuracy were a main effect of *group* $F(1;61) = 6.620$; $p = 0.013$, a main effect of *modality* $F(1;61) = 96.535$; $p < 0.001$ and an interaction effect *group × modality* $F(1;61) = 18.330$; $p < 0.001$, which means that participants with central facial paresis recognised visually presented basic emotions significantly worse (reduced accuracy) compared to participants without facial paresis ($t(49.425) = -3.767$; $p < 0.001$; after correction $p = 0.002$) and compared to healthy controls ($t(33) = -22.888$; $p < 0.001$; after correction $p = 0.002$). Participants without facial paresis recognised visually presented basic emotions significantly worse (reduced accuracy) compared to healthy controls ($t(28) = -10.476$; $p < 0.001$; after correction $p = 0.002$), Figure 1.

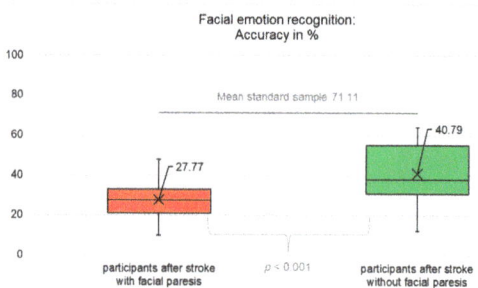

Figure 1. Accuracy of facial emotion recognition (mean, median, interquartile range). Participants after stroke with facial paresis performed significantly worse compared to healthy controls ($p < 0.001$) and compared to participants after stroke without facial paresis ($p < 0.001$). The data for healthy controls were not collected in this study but were taken from [46,47], so no information on the actual distribution of the data is available but only the mean as an indicator of the central tendency. Therefore, the figures only contain two box plots, not three.

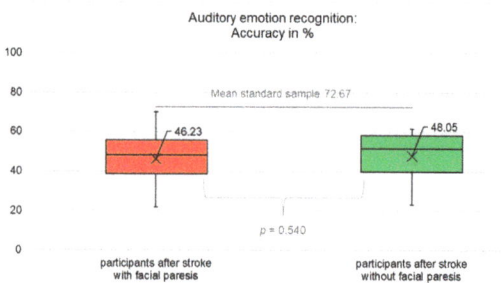

Figure 2. Accuracy of auditory emotion recognition (mean, median, interquartile range). Participants after stroke with facial paresis performed significantly worse compared to healthy controls ($p < 0.001$) but did not differ significantly compared to participants after stroke without facial paresis ($p = 0.540$). The data for healthy controls were not collected in this study but were taken from [45], so no information on the actual distribution of the data is available but only the mean as an indicator of the central tendency. Therefore, the figures only contain two box plots, not three.

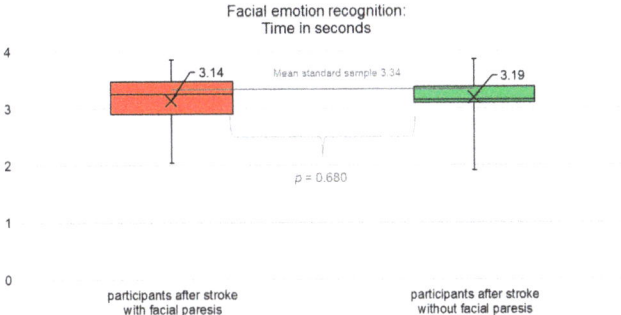

Figure 3. Average time of facial emotion recognition (mean, median, interquartile range). Participants after stroke with facial paresis performed significantly faster compared to healthy controls ($p = 0.02$) but did not differ significantly compared to participants after stroke without facial paresis ($p = 0.68$). The data for healthy controls were not collected in this study but were taken from [46,47], so no information on the actual distribution of the data is available but only the mean as an indicator of the central tendency. Therefore, the figures only contain two box plots, not three.

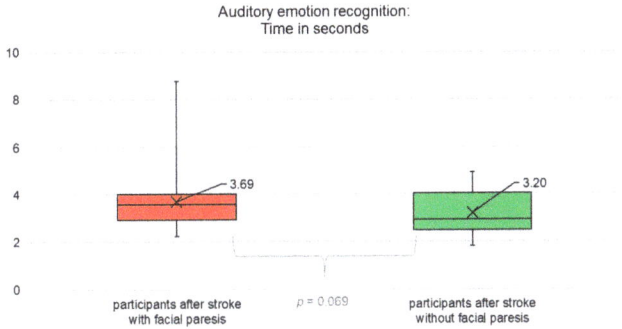

Figure 4. Average time taken for auditory emotion recognition (mean, median, interquartile range). Participants after stroke with facial paresis did not differ significantly compared to participants after stroke without facial paresis ($p = 0.069$).

3.2. Accuracy of Auditory Emotion Recognition

Participants with central facial paresis recognised auditorily presented basic emotions significantly worse (reduced accuracy) compared to healthy controls ($t(33) = -13.258$; $p < 0.001$; after correction $p = 0.002$). Participants without facial paresis recognised auditorily presented basic emotions significantly worse (reduced accuracy) compared to healthy controls ($t(28) = -11.259$; $p < 0.001$; after correction $p = 0.002$). Participants with vs. without central facial paresis did not differ significantly in auditory emotion recognition (accuracy) ($t(61) = 0.616$; $p = 0.540$; after correction $p = 0.540$), Figure 2.

3.3. Comparison of Accuracy of Facial and Auditory Emotion Recognition

Participants with central facial paresis recognised visually presented basic emotions significantly worse (reduced accuracy) than auditorily presented basic emotions ($t(33) =; -11252$; $p < 0.001$; after correction $p = 0.002$). Participants without facial paresis recognised visually presented basic emotions significantly worse (reduced accuracy) than auditorily presented basic emotions ($t(28) = -3.485$; $p = 0.002$; after correction $p = 0.002$).

3.4. Time Taken for Facial Emotion Recognition

The results of the ANOVA for accuracy were a main effect of *group* (F(1;61) = 2.797; $p = 0.100$), a main effect of *modality* (F(1;61) = 3.311; $p = 0.074$), and an interaction effect *group × modality* (F(1;61) = 3.148; $p = 0.081$)), which means that participants with central facial paresis did not recognise visually presented basic emotions significantly more slowly (reduced time) compared to participants without facial paresis (t(61) = 0.414; $p = 0.680$; after correction $p = 0.680$). Participants with central facial paresis recognised visually presented basic emotions significantly (not significantly after correction) faster (increased time) compared to healthy controls (t(33) = −2.442; $p = 0.020$; after correction $p = 0.060$). Participants without facial paresis recognised visually presented basic emotions significantly faster (increased time) compared to healthy controls (t(28) = −2.390; $p = 0.024$; after correction $p = 0.036$), Figure 3.

3.5. Time Taken for Auditory Emotion Recognition

Participants with vs. without central facial paresis did not differ significantly with respect to the average time taken for auditory emotion recognition (t(61) = −1.851; $p = 0.069$), Figure 4.

3.6. Comparison of Time Taken for Facial and Auditory Emotion Recognition

Participants with central facial paresis recognised visually presented basic emotions significantly (not significantly after correction) faster (increased time) than auditorily presented basic emotions (t(33) = −2.269; $p = 0.030$; after correction $p = 0.060$). Participants without facial paresis recognised visually presented basic emotions not significantly differently to auditorily presented basic emotions (t(28) = −0.041; $p = 0.968$; after correction $p = 0.968$).

3.7. Subjective Judgement of Emotion Recognition from the Perspective of Participants with Central Facial Paresis

Both the average accuracy of facial emotion recognition (mean = −0.71 ± 1.90) was perceived as significantly limited (t(33) = −2.167; $p = 0.038$; after correction $p = 0.038$) and the time taken for facial emotion recognition (mean = −1.91 ± 2.90) was subjectively perceived as significantly limited (t(33) = −3.849; $p = 0.001$; after correction $p = 0.003$) in participants with central facial paresis. Participants with central facial paresis judged themselves to be significantly more restricted in terms of the time taken for facial emotion recognition than in terms of accuracy (t(33) = 2.689; $p = 0.011$; after correction $p = 0.017$), Figure 5.

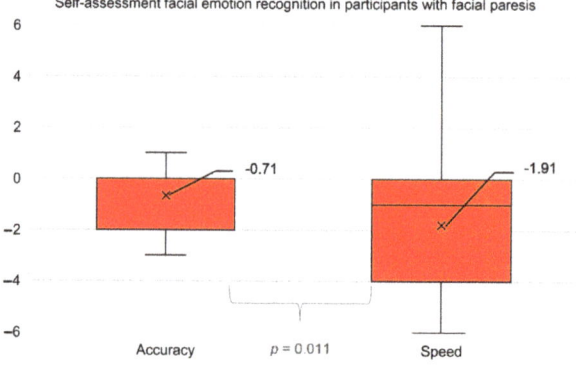

Figure 5. Accuracy and time taken in subjective facial emotion recognition (mean, median, interquartile range) in participants after stroke with facial paresis. Participants felt significantly more restricted in terms of time compared to accuracy ($p = 0.011$).

3.8. Further Analysis

In order to verify that the identified pattern is reasonable on the basis of these results, the following further control calculations were made.

A correlation calculation (Pearson's product moment correlation) between objective accuracy and objective time taken for facial emotion recognition in patients with and without central facial paresis was performed. The accuracy of and the time taken for facial emotion recognition in patients with central facial paresis were positively correlated with each other ($r = 0.729$; $p < 0.001$). The average accuracy and the average time taken for facial emotion recognition in patients without facial paresis were not significantly correlated with each other ($r = 0.291$; $p = 0.126$).

Furthermore, a correlation calculation (Pearson's product moment correlation) between objective facial emotion recognition, accuracy and severity of facial paresis using the Sunnybrook Facial Grading System across all patients (with and without facial paresis) was performed. The average accuracy of facial emotion recognition and the severity of facial paresis were significantly positively correlated with each other ($r = 0.31$; $p = 0.014$).

Moreover, a one-tailed *t*-test on independent samples for facial emotion recognition accuracy showed no significant difference between patients with left-sided facial paresis (mean = 26.44 ± 11.49) and right-sided facial paresis (mean = 29.25 ± 10.69), $t(32) = -0.734$; $p = 0.234$. Another one tailed *t*-test on independent samples for facial emotion recognition time showed no significant difference between patients with left-sided facial paresis (mean = 3.12 ± 0.48) and right-sided facial paresis (mean = 3.17 ± 0.47), $t(32) = -0.322$; $p = 0.375$.

Furthermore, a chi-squared test to compare the number of patients with limitations in general mental capacity in both groups (Table A5, Appendix A) was performed. Both groups were comparable, with $x^2(1, n = 63) = 0.204$; $p = 0.651$. Another chi-squared test to compare the number of patients with aphasia in both groups (Table A6, Appendix A) was also carried out. Both groups were comparable, with $x^2(1, n = 63) = 1.546$; $p = 0.214$.

Additionally, univariate and multivariate regressions, with emotion recognition (facial and auditory, accuracy and time taken) as the dependent variable and predictors diagnosis of facial paresis, sex, age, subjective judgement, general mental capacity and time post-onset as independent variables, were conducted (Tables A7 and A8, Appendix A). Patients with facial paresis recognised visually presented basic emotions significantly worse (reduced accuracy) compared to patients without facial paresis, as calculated by means of univariate regression (beta = -0.444; $p < 0.001$) as well as by multivariate regression (beta = -0.353; 0.003).

4. Discussion

This study investigated visual facial emotion recognition (VFER) in patients with and without central facial paresis vs. healthy individuals. The results of our study showed that the participants with central facial paresis had significantly lower average accurate emotion recognition abilities with respect to the facial modality compared to the auditory modality. The less accurate VFER in cases of facial paresis but not in auditory emotion recognition may be due to changes in the facial feedback mechanism. Clinically, this means that VFER in persons with limited facial mimicry abilities, as in central facial paresis patients, does appear to be affected, in contrast to auditory recognition [36]. Taking into account that we did not test facial mimicry itself (i.e., facial muscle activity was not measured during the emotion-recognition task), but facial emotion recognition, facial paresis can be inferred to be one factor influencing the accuracy of objective facial emotion recognition, which may be affected by changes in the facial feedback mechanism. This may be an indication that the accuracy of objective facial emotion recognition is especially limited when facial feedback is altered by facial paresis. Auditory performance does not appear to be affected by facial paresis (for a similar finding, cf. [36]). Besides facial paresis, stroke, also, could be one factor influencing the accuracy of objective facial emotion recognition in our sample. All participants (with and without facial paresis) had had at least one stroke. Since stroke may also cause deficits in emotion recognition [43], our examined patient groups may be affected as well. These two potential factors (altered facial feedback and altered central processing due to stroke) indicate the relevance of and need to study patients without stroke but with limited facial feedback—for example, patients with peripheral facial palsy.

Our results reveal significant deficits in terms of accuracy of facial emotion recognition, in contrast with other studies that did not report any differences, e.g., [27,28,34]. This fact may be due to the large sample size (participants with facial paresis: n = 34; participants without facial paresis: n = 29) and the inclusion of different phases post-onset, with a wide range since the time of stroke (day 5 up to day 6361 post-onset). However, previous studies reported significant limitations in terms of average time taken for facial emotion recognition, e.g., [27,28], while the participants in the present study showed faster reaction times. This, in turn, could indicate that the participants after stroke replied *quick and dirty* [63], while they suffered from other impairments, such as deficits in attention, concentration and memory [64], in addition to the facial paresis after stroke. In order to investigate a possible systemic connection between the fast, inaccurate responses, the significant positive correlation between the objective accuracy and the objective time taken for facial emotion recognition in patients with facial paresis provides further insight: the faster a patient with facial paresis responded, the less accurate was the response, whereas no correlation was found in patients without facial paresis. This could indicate that the patients with facial paresis were themselves aware of their deficit in the time taken for facial emotion recognition (as reported in the *Self-Assessment Questionnaires Emotion Recognition*) but wanted to show their best performance in the test situation and therefore answered as quickly as possible.

The participants with facial paresis subjectively felt limited both in terms of parameter accuracy and time in VFER. They stated that they were more impaired with respect to time than accuracy. The participants felt that facial emotion recognition had slowed down considerably since the stroke and was somewhat less accurate. These results provide a new insight into subjective emotion recognition, as this was not considered in previous studies. However, the clinical measurement gave contradictory results and showed that the patients were clearly less accurate but faster. Thus, the measured performance appears to be controversial to the subjectively perceived performance.

In the present study, we considered the difference in facial and auditory emotion recognition shown in the results. This may support, for example, FFH, as mentioned before. Nevertheless, it should be noted that a large part of human emotion is communicated via the face *and* the voice, as discussed in the literature. To the best of our knowledge, this is the first clinical study which combines two different modalities in a clinical setting [65]. The mentioned factors (limitations such as deficits in attention, concentration and memory [64], besides facial paresis and emotion recognition) influenced both the study results and everyday communication in the patient groups. Although for stroke patients their survival is of primary importance [66], participation is also highly relevant, particularly in the post-acute and chronic phase [67]. Since both groups of patients showed a significant reduction in the accuracy of facial and auditory emotion recognition compared to healthy subjects, intervention recommendations for both groups and both modalities are required. Although there is limited evidence for FFH [68], FFH can be used as an explanation for assessment and rehabilitation [69].

4.1. The Relevance of Assessment of Emotion Recognition

The described results not only provide evidence for the FFH and certain effects of stroke but also have implications for the treatment of patients with central facial paresis after stroke. As early as 2013, Dobel et al. [69] called for the examination of facial emotion recognition in patients with facial paresis using basic emotions [69]. In summary, the present study supports this demand and once again advocates it.

Since the accuracy of facial emotion recognition can be impaired, especially in patients with facial paresis after stroke, appropriate assessment and therapy is recommended for this patient group. Deficits should be assessed because the performance limitations may have negative consequences on communication and may increase over time. If the performance of emotion recognition remains impaired, this can lead to the development of disorders such as alexithymia (the inability to recognise or describe one's own emotions) [11,70]. For example, if sadness is not adequately interpreted, a patient may react defensively and thus not appropriately to a situation [6]. The effects of facial emotion recognition are therefore far-reaching and decisive for adequate social contact. The somewhat controversial results for the objective measurement and subjective assessment of facial emotion recognition in participants with facial paresis require detailed and individual examination in clinical practice. It is not sufficient to *either* ask the patient for his or her opinion *or* carry out an objective diagnosis. Both options should be taken and the results should be compared.

In addition, the lack of disease insight to be expected according to the available results (comparison between clinical measurement and subjective assessment) must become a focus of treatment in order to show the patient the relevance of facial emotion recognition therapy. This should not underestimate the importance of considering the individual wishes and goals of the patient and including them in the sense of joint decision making [71]. The basis for this is the tripartite evidence-based practice [71,72]. This ensures not only the effectiveness and efficiency of therapy, but also therapy motivation and transfer into the patient's everyday life [71].

4.2. Limitations of the Study

The composition of the sample may be considered a limiting factor of the study. A larger and more representative, homogeneous sample tested at the same time post-onset after stroke and subdivided according to the subtypes of central facial paresis (voluntary and involuntary central facial paresis [73]) would therefore be desirable for future studies. For a more precise observation of the lesion localization and comparability of patients, imaging with detailed description of affected brain areas would be useful. In addition, statistical adjustment for different stroke locations and lesion sizes would be beneficial, as differences in emotion recognition could depend on the hemisphere affected [43]. Despite the possibility of different lesion locations and lesion sizes, the results for facial emotion recognition showed significant differences between the patient groups. Since significant effects can already be observed in our sample, we expect similar or stronger effects to be observed with more carefully selected samples with stricter inclusion criteria in further studies. Furthermore, a strong and reliable test battery to assess cognitive capacity (see [74]) is needed to differentiate deficits in emotion recognition and limitations on general mental capacity after stroke. Since emotion perception depends on general mental capacity [74–76], any emotion perception test measures general mental capacity to some degree. In the present study, there were comparable numbers of patients with limitations in mental capacity and aphasia, as proven by chi-squared tests. In future studies, comparability should be extended and improved by standardised diagnostics.

However, the significant positive correlation observed between objective facial emotion recognition accuracy and severity of facial paresis, calculated using the *Sunnybrook Facial Grading System* across all patients, points to facial paresis as the main differentiator between the two patient groups. Thus, the higher the accuracy of facial emotion recognition, the higher the score on the *Sunnybrook Facial Grading System*. That is, facial competence correlates with accuracy in facial emotion recognition, or the lower the facial competence, the worse the accuracy in facial emotion recognition. Moreover, significant univariate and multivariate regressions documented the relation between facial emotion recognition accuracy and facial paresis. These results demonstrate the influence of facial paresis on facial emotion recognition once more, but only in terms of accuracy. No significant differences were detected with respect to objective facial emotion recognition accuracy and time taken between patients with left- or right-sided facial paresis. If one hemisphere is dominant in emotion processing [43], patients with lesions in this dominant hemisphere with contralateral facial paresis [25] could possibly be more affected. We cannot confirm this hypothesis and previous research on facial palsy that reported that patients with left-sided facial palsy showed lower performance in facial emotion recognition compared with patients with right-sided facial palsy [29]. However, our results are in line with findings for patients with Parkinson's disease, where facial asymmetry is not related to hemispheric dominance for emotion processing [77]. Further evidence is needed, then, to inspect possible differences in facial emotion recognition and expression depending on the side affected with facial palsy and on hemisphere.

Perfect comparability of the standard data with the sample data cannot be guaranteed without gaps—for instance, due to the age of the participants (e.g., the *Montreal Affective Voices* validation sample with an average age of 23.3 ± 3 years [45] vs. the patients with facial paresis with an average age of 62.6 ± 9.3 years and patients without facial paresis average with an average age of 58.4 ± 10.7 years). It must also be noted that only a small sample size of normative data (n = 29) was used for the auditory emotion recognition assessment *(Montreal Affective Voices)* [45]. Furthermore, the measurement of auditory and facial emotion recognition is not completely comparable. Especially with regard to the time taken for emotion recognition, it should be noted, for example, that the response modes differed (selecting an option on screen vs. pointing to a surface) and that the numbers of items and response options were not identical. As a consequence, for further research, normative data from healthy individuals should be freshly collected, with comparability extended to the patient groups. Moreover, measurement in facial and auditory emotion recognition tasks should be made even more comparable.

The separate presentation of facial and auditory items in emotion recognition assessments should also be critically questioned. Facial and auditory expressions are not necessarily independent as they can mutually influence their recognition. For example, a facial expression can be generated by moving the mouth while a vocal expression is also made [1]. However, a separation of the modalities, i.e., just visual or just auditory impressions, seemed to make sense in this study in order to differentiate and compare performances. In order to be able to answer the question reliably, this seems unavoidable. At the same time, however, this separate type of emotion recognition is far removed from everyday life and thus reduces the external validity. Equally adapted to optimal experimental conditions, static photographs instead of everyday situations were used [78]. A person is able to show up to 8000 different emotional facial expressions with his or her face [17]. However, it should be critically noted that our study only examined emotion recognition with respect to basic emotions and thus minimized the requirements compared to non-verbal communication in everyday life. It should be noted here that basic emotions can be regarded as the basis for far more complex emotions or emotional states [8]. However, since the recognition of the comparatively primitive basic emotions [8] was assessed as limited in the present study, an even worse performance can be expected for more complex emotions.

5. Conclusions

From this study, it may be concluded that:
- After a stroke, participants with central facial paresis were significantly less accurate in visually recognising basic emotions compared with stroke patients without facial paresis and compared with a sample of healthy controls;
- Auditory emotion recognition in both stroke groups was less accurate than in the control sample;
- The facial emotion recognition accuracy of participants with central facial paresis was significantly worse than the auditory accuracy of emotion recognition;
- Since visual emotion recognition was clearly worse than auditory emotion recognition in participants with facial paresis after stroke, facial mimicry probably plays an important role in communication with patients after stroke;

- The results of our observational study may indicate the overall effects of stroke on emotion recognition and support the FFH, which is a practical and appropriate model implemented in clinical assessments and interventions;
- Future research should investigate patients with facial palsy without stroke to further explore the impact of facial feedback on emotion recognition.

Author Contributions: Conceptualization, A.-M.K., H.v.P. and S.H.; methodology, A.-M.K., H.v.P. and S.H.; software, A.-M.K.; validation, A.-M.K.; formal analysis, A.-M.K. and S.H.; investigation, A.-M.K.; resources, A.-M.K., H.v.P. and S.H.; data curation, A.-M.K. and S.H.; writing—original draft preparation, A.-M.K.; writing—review and editing, A.-M.K., H.v.P. and S.H.; visualization, A.-M.K.; supervision, H.v.P. and S.H.; project administration, A.-M.K.; funding acquisition A.-M.K. All authors have read and agreed to the published version of the manuscript.

Funding: The APC was funded by Thüringer Universitäts- und Landesbibliothek Jena, Germany.

Institutional Review Board Statement: All subjects gave their informed consent for inclusion before they participated in the study. The study was conducted according to the guidelines of the Declaration of Helsinki, and the protocol was approved by the Ethics Committee of the Medical Faculty at RWTH Aachen University, Germany (protocol code: EK 271/18; 11 December 2018).

Informed Consent Statement: Informed consent was obtained from all subjects involved in the study.

Data Availability Statement: The data presented in this study are available on request from the corresponding author. The data are not publicly available due to their having been collected as part of a larger research project that has not yet been completed.

Acknowledgments: Many thanks to all of the study participants and cooperation partners: Berufsfachschule für Logopädie an der staatlichen berufsbildenden Schule für Gesundheit und Soziales Jena, Klinikum Ingolstadt GmbH, Logopädie Sprechfreude, Dasing, Moritz Klinik GmbH & Co. KG, Bad Klosterlausnitz, Praxis für Sprach- und Stimmtherapie Hermine Gascho, Ingolstadt, Selbsthilfegruppe Aphasiker und Schlaganfall Jena des Landesverbandes Thüringen für die Rehabilitation der Aphasiker e. V., Beratungszentrum nach Schlaganfall und Hirnschädigung ZAMOR e. V. Ingolstadt and Uniklinik RWTH Aachen AöR.

Conflicts of Interest: The authors declare no conflict of interest.

Appendix A

Table A1. Sociodemographic information on gender, age, education and handedness in the study group and control groups.

Sociodemographic Information	Study Group Patients with Facial Paresis, n = 34	Control Group Patients without Facial Paresis, n = 29
Gender	Male: n = 18; 53% Female: n = 16; 47%	Male: n = 20; 69% Female: n = 9; 31%
Age in years	Mean = 62.65 ± 9.26 Min. = 39 Max. = 81	Mean = 58.38 ± 10.72 Min. = 35 Max. = 83
Education	No school degree: n = 4; 11.77% Sec. school certificate: n = 9; 26.47% Medium maturity: n = 12; 35.29% High school: n = 9; 26.47%	No school degree: n = 0 Sec. school certificate: n = 6; 20.69% Medium maturity: n = 15; 51.72% High school: n = 8; 27.59%
Handedness	Left: n = 0 Right: n = 33; 97.06% Left and right: n = 1; 2.94%	Left: n = 1. 3.45% Right: n = 27; 93.10% Left and right: n = 1; 3.45%

Note: n = number of participants.

Table A2. Lesion information, times post-onset of the examinations in this study, type of lesion (ischaemic, hemorrhagic or both), affected hemisphere, quantity (number of lesions), limitations in general mental capacity after stroke and aphasia.

Lesion	Study Group Patients with Facial Paresis, n = 34	Control Group Patients without Facial Paresis, n = 29
Time post-onset in days (in years;months)	Mean = 1558 (4;3) ± 2112 (5;9) Min. = 5 Max. = 6361 (17;5)	Mean = 1359 (3;9) ± 2702 (7;5) Min. = 13 Max. = 11,398 (31;2)
Phase post-onset (Acute: ≤6 weeks Post-acute: <1 year Chronic: ≥1 year)	Acute: n = 11; 32.35% Post-acute: n = 6; 17.65% Chronic: n = 17; 50.00%	Acute: n = 11; 37.93% Post-acute: n = 3; 10.34% Chronic: n = 15; 51.72%
Type	Ischemic: n = 27; 79.41% Hemorrhagic: n = 5; 14.71% Ischemic and hemorrhagic: n = 1; 2.94% n.a.: n = 1; 2.94%	Ischemic: n = 21; 72.41% Hemorrhagic: n = 6; 20.69% Ischemic and hemorrhagic: n = 1; 3.45% n.a.: n = 1; 3.45%
Hemisphere	Left: n = 12; 35.29% Right: n = 13; 38.24% Left and right: n = 0 n.a.: n = 9; 26.47%	Left: n = 15; 51.72% Right: n = 6; 20.69% Left and right: n = 2; 6.90% n.a.: n = 6; 20.69%
Quantity	1x: n = 22; 64.71% 2x: n = 8; 23.53% 3x: n = 1; 2.94% 4x: n = 1; 2.94% n.a.: n = 2; 5.88%	1x: n = 25; 86.21% 2x: n = 2; 6.90% 3x: n = 1; 3.45% 4x: n = 0 n.a.: n = 1; 3.45%
Limitations in general mental capacity after stroke	n = 16; 47.06%	n = 12; 41.38%
Aphasia	n = 6; 17.65%	n = 9; 31.03%

Note: n.a. means no information was given. n = number of participants.

Table A3. Facial paresis information; diagnosis from the patients' perspectives and from the patients' therapists' perspectives, according to the participant; diagnosis via Sunnybrook Facial Grading System [52,53] carried out as part of this study by a logopaedic examiner and severity classification according to the House–Brackmann Facial Nerve Grading System [79], as well as affected side of the face, time post-onset of the examination for this study and already perceived therapy prior to examination in this study.

Facial Paresis	Study Group Patients with Facial Paresis, n = 34	Control Group Patients without Facial Paresis, n = 29
Diagnosis facial paresis from the patient's perspective	Facial paresis: n = 21; 61.76% - Left: n = 9; 26.47% - Right: n = 12; 35.29% Non-facial paresis: n = 13; 38.24%	Facial paresis: n = 10; 34.48% - Left: n = 2; 6.90% - Right: n = 8; 27.58% Non-facial paresis: n = 19; 65.52%
Diagnosis of facial paresis from the therapist's perspective (physiotherapy or speech and language therapy)	Facial paresis: n = 11; 32.35% - Left: n = 4; 11.76% - Right: n = 6; 17.65% - n.a. to the affected side: n = 1; 2.94% Non-facial paresis: n = 2; 5.88% n.a.: n = 21; 61.77%	Facial paresis: n = 0 Non-facial paresis: n = 6; 20.69% n.a.: n = 23; 79.31%

Table A3. Cont.

Facial Paresis	Study Group Patients with Facial Paresis, n = 34	Control Group Patients without Facial Paresis, n = 29
Diagnosis of facial paresis *Sunnybrook Facial Grading System* (total score 0–100)	Mean = 73.12 ± 8.34 Min. = 54 Max. = 83 Grade II: n = 24; 70.59% Grade III: n = 10; 29.41% Left: - Grade II: n = 11; 61.11% - Grade III: n = 7; 38.89% Right: - Grade II: n = 13; 81.25% - Grade III: n = 3; 18.75%	Mean = 91.21 ± 3.46 Min. = 87 Max. = 100 Grade I: n = 29; 100%
Time post-onset in days (in years;months)	Mean = 827 (2;3) ± 1606 (4;5) Min. = 5 Max. = 5852 (16;0)	Mean = 2207 (6;1) ±3709 (10;2) Min. = 35 Max. = 11,398 (31;2)
Phase post-onset (Acute: ≤6 weeks Post-acute: <1 year Chronic: ≥1 year)	Acute: n = 14; 41.18% Post-acute: n = 5; 14.71% Chronic: n = 7; 20.59% n.a.: n = 8; 23.53%	Acute: n = 3; 10.35% Post-acute: n = 1; 3.45% Chronic: n = 9; 31.03% n.a.: n = 16; 55.17%
Non-pharmaceutical therapy at the time of the examination (current)	Yes: n = 9; 26.47% No: n = 25; 73.53%	Yes: n = 0 No: n = 29
Start	From the stroke to latest post-acute phase	From the stroke to latest post-acute phase
Frequency	Isolated therapy units up to 1–3x/week	Individual therapy units up to 2x/week
Duration	Max.: 3.5 months	Max.: 6 months
Therapist	12x speech and language therapy, 2x physiotherapy, 1x physical therapy	5x speech and language therapy, 1x physiotherapy, 1x n.a.
Content	Exercises for facial expression, oral motor skills, articulation, proprioceptive neuromuscular facilitation, massage	Exercises for facial expression, oral motor skills, articulation, stretching M. buccinator
Self-exercises	Exercises for facial expression, oral motor skills, articulation, massage, sensitivity training	Exercises for facial expressions, oral motor skills

Note: n.a. means no information was given. n = number of participants.

Table A4. The results for objective (accuracy and time) and subjectively perceived success in emotion recognition are summarised.

Emotion Recognition	Study Group Patients with Facial Paresis, n = 34	Control Group Patients without Facial Paresis, n = 29	Healthy Controls
Objective facial emotion recognition via *Myfacetraining* Programm, Accuracy in %	Mean = 27.77 SD = 11.04 Min. = 10.00 Max. = 48.00	Mean = 40.79 SD = 15.59 Min. = 12.00 Max. = 64.00	Mean = 71.11 SD = 7.53 Min. = 45.00 Max. = 88.00 n = 147 [46,47]
Objective facial emotion recognition via *Myfacetraining* Program, Time in sec.	Mean = 3.14 SD = 0.47 Min. = 2.04 Max. = 3.86	Mean = 3.19 SD = 0.34 Min. = 1.91 Max. = 3.86	Mean = 3.34 SD = 0.66 Min. = 1.94 Max. = 5.58 n = 147 [46,47]
Objective auditory emotion recognition via *MAVs*, Accuracy in %	Mean = 46.23 SD = 11.63 Min. = 21.67 Max. = 70.00	Mean = 48.05 SD = 11.78 Min. = 23.34 Max. = 61.67	Mean = 72.67 SD = 11.99 Min. = 56.00 Max. = 86.00 n = 29 [45]
Objective auditory emotion recognition via *MAVs*, Time in sec.	Mean = 3.69 SD = 1.20 Min. = 2.25 Max. = 8.75	Mean = 3.20 SD = 0.88 Min. = 1.80 Max. = 4.90	n.a. [45]
Subjective facial emotion recognition via *Self-Assessment Questionnaires* Emotion Recognition Accuracy	Mean = −0.71 SD = 1.90 Min. = −6.00 Max. = 6.00	Mean = −0.03 SD = 1.32 Min. = −2.00 Max. = 6.00	n.a.
Subjective facial emotion recognition via *Self-Assessment Questionnaires* Emotion Recognition Time	Mean = −1.91 SD = 2.90 Min. = −6.00 Max. = 6.00	Mean = −1.00 SD = 2.52 Min. = −6.00 Max. = 6.00	n.a.

Note: n.a. means no information was given. n = number of participants.

Table A5. Summary of facial paresis and general mental capacity information.

	Study Group Patients with Facial Paresis, n = 34	Control Group Patients without Facial Paresis, n = 29
With limitations in general mental capacity	n = 16	n = 12
Without limitations in general mental capacity	n = 18	n = 17
Types of limitation in general mental capacity	Memory: n = 10 Concentration: n = 9 Slowdown: n = 3 Fatigue: n = 2 Complex thinking: n = 1 Neglect on spec: n = 1 Orientation in time: n = 1 Orientation in place: n = 1 Overall deterioration: n = 1 Acalculia: n = 0 Arousal: n = 0 Inner unrest: n = 0	Memory: n = 8 Concentration: n = 5 Slowdown: n = 1 Fatigue: n = 2 Complex thinking: n = 0 Neglect on spec: n = 0 Orientation in time: n = 0 Orientation in place: n = 0 Overall deterioration: n = 0 Acalculia: n = 1 Arousal: n = 1 Inner unrest: n = 1

Note: n = number of participants. For limitations in general mental capacity, multiple deficit types per participant are possible. For this, n describes the number of limitations per group.

Table A6. Summary of facial paresis and aphasia information.

	Study Group Patients with Facial Paresis, n = 34	Control Group Patients without Facial Paresis, n = 29
With aphasia	n = 6	n = 9
Without aphasia	n = 28	n = 20

Note: n = number of participants.

Table A7. Univariate regression analysis.

	Accuracy of Facial Emotion Recognition			
	Standardised Beta	95.0% Confidence Interval		p-Value
		Lower bound	Higher bound	
Diagnosis of facial paresis	−0.444	−19.762	−6.295	<0.001
	Time taken for facial emotion recognition			
Diagnosis of facial paresis	−0.053	−0.253	0.166	0.680
	Accuracy of auditory emotion recognition			
Diagnosis of facial paresis	−0.079	−7.733	4.091	0.540
	Time taken for auditory emotion recognition			
Diagnosis of facial paresis	0.231	−0.040	1.033	0.069

Table A8. Multivariate regression analysis.

	Accuracy of Facial Emotion Recognition			
	Standardised Beta	95.0% Confidence Interval		p-Value
		Lower bound	Higher bound	
Diagnosis of facial paresis	−0.353	−16.920	−3.787	0.003
Sex	0.022	−6.306	7.615	0.851
Age	−0.393	−0.891	−0.256	<0.001
Subjective judgement of accuracy	−0.014	−2.359	2.110	0.911
Subjective judgement of time taken	0.032	−1.197	1.542	0.802
Limitations in general mental capacity	0.054	−5.213	8.392	0.641
Time post-onset, acute, post-acute, chronic	−0.227	−7.417	0.128	0.058
	Time of facial emotion recognition			
Diagnosis of facial paresis	−0.029	−0.248	0.201	0.834
Sex	−0.173	−0.383	0.093	0.228
Age	−0.186	−0.018	0.003	0.167
Subjective judgement of accuracy	0.013	−0.073	0.080	0.935
Subjective judgement of time taken	0.057	−0.038	0.055	0.715
Limitations in general mental capacity	0.076	−0.170	0.295	0.593
Time post-onset, acute, post-acute, chronic	−0.252	−0.242	0.016	0.085

Table A8. Cont.

	Accuracy of Facial Emotion Recognition			
	Standardised Beta	95.0% Confidence Interval		p-Value
	Accuracy of auditory emotion recognition			
Diagnosis of facial paresis	0.015	−4.900	5.596	0.895
Sex	0.082	−3.638	7.488	0.491
Age	−0.428	−0.747	−0.239	<0.001
Subjective judgement of accuracy	−0.160	−2.894	0.678	0.219
Subjective judgement of time taken	0.106	−0.646	1.542	0.416
Limitations in general mental capacity	0.068	−3.859	7.015	0.563
Time post-onset, acute, post-acute, chronic	−0.374	−7.750	−1.720	0.003
	Time of auditory emotion recognition			
Diagnosis of facial paresis	0.227	−0.074	1.052	0.088
Sex	−0.050	−0.706	0.489	0.717
Age	0.153	−0.011	0.044	0.232
Subjective judgement of accuracy	0.184	−0.073	0.310	0.220
Subjective judgement of time taken	−0.033	−0.131	0.104	0.825
Limitations in general mental capacity	−0.173	−0.959	0.209	0.203
Time post-onset, acute, post-acute, chronic	0.205	−0.083	0.565	0.141

Appendix B

Appendix B.1 Additional Information on Data Collection

Each patient was examined once. The patient was first informed about the study and about data privacy. After the declaration of informed consent, an anamnesis took place (see Tables A1–A3, Appendix A) before the examination was conducted. All data were collected by the same examiner. All participants received the same standardised verbal instruction to perform the following tasks.

Appendix B.2 Facial Emotion Recognition: Myfacetraining (MFT) Program

The *Myfacetraining* (MFT) Program (CRAFTA Cranio Facial Therapy Academy, Hamburg, Germany) [47,49] measured objective facial emotion recognition with respect to accuracy and time taken [47,49]. Portraits of people, each showing a basic emotion with their face, were presented on a *lenovo yoga 500* 14″ touchscreen device. The person was first shown in a neutral position (one second) then with an emotional facial expression (basic emotion). Six additional answer options were displayed on the right side of the screen; these were the basic emotions [47].

By selecting an answer option (in 85% (n = 54) of cases via touchscreen, in 6.35% (n = 4) of cases via touch-pen due to hemiparesis, in 7.95% (n = 5) via mouse due to hemiparesis), the program recorded the accuracy (right or wrong answer) as well as the reaction time (in seconds). Immediately afterwards, the next screen appeared. In a standardised test, a total of 42 images of three different adult women and three different men (one person per picture) in the same order were presented. Each basic emotion was shown seven times (six basic emotions × seven images = 42 images). The time limit to respond was 10 s. If there was no response within this time, the response time was considered to have been exceeded and therefore the question was marked *unanswered* and the next emotion was presented. Objective facial emotion recognition was measured with respect to accuracy and time [47]. After testing, the program reproduced an overview of the time taken and the accuracy scores for all the emotion questions together and separately and the time and exchange emotion, if available, for all 42 pictures.

A pre-test with ten items was performed. The pre-test ensured that the task was understood [48]. Questions asked of the patient regarding the test procedure were answered. However, no assistance was given with regard to the content of the test.

With the *Myfacetraining* Program, normal values for 147 healthy subjects are available. Accuracy in percentages: mean = 71.11 ± 7.53; min. = 45.00; max. = 88.00. Time in seconds: mean = 3.34 ± 0.66; min. = 1.94; max. = 5.58 [46,47] (see, also, Figures 1 and 3; Table A4, Appendix A).

Appendix B.3 Auditory Emotion Recognition: Montreal Affective Voices

As stimuli for auditory emotion recognition, part of the *Montreal Affective Voices* (*MAVs*) [45] was used. These are emotional, non-linguistic, vocal expressions of /a/ (to be compared with a as in *apple*, British English). Five women and five men each presented the six basic emotions with their voice once each [45], so that in the present study a total of 60 (= 10 persons × 6 basic emotions) items were used.

For the presentation of the *MAVs*, software was available which, in addition to the accuracy of emotion recognition, also checks the intensity of the emotion but neglects the time taken [80]. For the present study, which examined the accuracy and time taken for emotion recognition, the procedure had therefore to be adapted. For this purpose, a specially programmed experiment with the software *PsychoPy*, version 3.0.0b9 [50] was used, which on the one hand reproduced the *MAVs* and on the other hand recorded the selected response option and reaction time. The sound was given once [80] via standard headphones [45]. The sequence of stimuli was randomised and standardised and presented in the same order for all participants.

Each participant was asked to assess an emotion by selecting a response option [81]. Following the original software [80], the participant selected one of the response options (one of the six basic emotions or *neutral/unknown*) by pointing at a surface (A4 size). Ten seconds of time were allowed for response to each task.

As in objective facial emotion recognition, a pre-test with ten items (initially randomised, later presented in the same order) was performed too. In addition, the examiner checked that the headphones were comfortably fitted. The volume was adjusted individually [45]. Questions asked of the patient regarding the test procedure were answered. However, no assistance was given with regard to the content of the test.

Standard values are available for accuracy (in percentages) of emotion recognition: mean = 72,67 ± 11.66; min. = 56.00; max. = 86.00 (see, also, Figure 2 and Table A4, Appendix A). However, no data were collected for time taken [45]. As proposed by Belin et al. [45] and explained above, *MAVs* (selected items, adapted to the circumstances of this study) were used. The *MAVs*, as material for auditory emotion recognition assessment, are explicitly recommended for comparisons of facial emotion recognition. They are particularly well-suited, since only the auditory modality is addressed. Furthermore, the *MAVs* do not contain any linguistic information, which excludes distortion or aggravated conditions for patients with aphasia [45]. Mild aphasia was not necessarily a criterion for exclusion in this study (see Table 1).

Appendix B.4 Sunnybrook Facial Grading System for Diagnosing Facial Palsy

With the *Sunnybrook Facial Grading System*, each face was rated in three areas by comparing the affected side of the face with the intact side. This resulted in three values: (1) *Resting Symmetry Score* (symmetry at rest), (2) *Voluntary Movement Score* (symmetry of voluntary movements) and (3) *Synkinesis Score* (synkinesis). With these three scores, a *total score* (0–100 points) was calculated. The lower the *total score*, the more pronounced the facial paresis respectively paralysis. The authors did not give any recommendation for a further classification according to degree of severity or the point value for a diagnosis of *facial palsy* actually made [52,53]. For the present study, however, an unambiguous diagnosis of the presence of facial paresis seemed indispensable to classify the participants into the appropriate target or control groups (with or without facial paresis). The severity classification of the present study was therefore based on the procedures of the *House–Brackman Facial Nerve Grading System* [79] and the *Facial Nerve Grading System 2.0* [55]. For these measuring instruments, the total value to be achieved is divided into six groups or grades (degree I: normal function up to degree VI: total paralysis) [55,79]. This classification was also used in the present work. For this purpose, the maximum *total score* (100 points) to be achieved in the *Sunnybrook Facial Grading System* was divided by six and thus into six equally sized areas (100–84 points: normal function, no facial paresis; 83–67: light facial paresis; 66–50 moderate facial paresis; 49–33 medium facial paresis; 32–16 severe facial paresis; 15–0 complete facial paresis with respect to paralysis). Once the *total score* had been evaluated by the logopaedic examiner, the severity level could be determined. According to this definition, a facial paresis from grade II ($\leq$83 points) could be presented. This, in turn, implied an admission of a natural portion of asymmetry in the face and is consistent with previous research [82].

References

1. Schirmer, A.; Adolphs, R. Emotion Perception from Face, Voice, and Touch: Comparisons and Convergence. *Trends Cogn. Sci.* **2017**, *21*, 216–228. [CrossRef] [PubMed]
2. Young, A.; Perrett, D.; Calder, A.; Sprengelmeyer, R.; Ekman, P. *Facial Expressions of Emotion—Stimuli and Tests (FEEST)*; Thames Valley Test Company: Suffolk, UK, 2002.
3. Knapp, M.L.; Hall, J.A.; Horgan, T.G. *Nonverbal Communication in Human Interaction*; Cengage Learning: Boston, MA, USA, 2013.
4. Ekman, P.; Oster, H. Facial Expression of Emotion. *Annu. Rev. Psychol.* **1979**, *30*, 527–554. [CrossRef]
5. Diener, H.C. 2016. Available online: https://www.pschyrembel.de/Parese/K0GCP/doc/ (accessed on 25 June 2020).
6. Radice-Neumann, D.; Zupan, B.; Tomita, M.; Willer, B. Training Emotional Processing in Persons With Brain Injury. *J. Head Trauma Rehabil.* **2009**, *5*, 313–323. [CrossRef] [PubMed]

7. Cattaneo, L.; Pavesi, G. The facial motor system. *Neurosci. Biobehav. Rev.* **2014**, *38*, 135–159. [CrossRef]
8. Levenson, R.W. Basic Emotion Questions. *Emot. Rev.* **2011**, *3*, 379–386. [CrossRef]
9. Ekman, P. Universal Facial Expressions of Emotion. *Calif. Ment. Health Res. Dig.* **1970**, *8*, 151–158.
10. Ekman, P. An argument for basic emotions. *Cogn. Emot.* **1992**, *6*, 169–200. [CrossRef]
11. Dimberg, U.; Thunberg, M.; Elmehed, K. Unconscious Facial Reactions to Emotional Facial Expressions. *Psychol. Sci.* **2000**, *11*, 86–89. [CrossRef]
12. Boloorizadeh, P.; Tojari, F. Facial expression recognition: Age, gender and exposure duration impact. *Pro-Cedia Soc. Behav. Sci.* **2013**, *84*, 1369–1375. [CrossRef]
13. Williams, L.M.; Mathersul, D.; Palmer, D.M.; Gur, R.C.; Gur, R.E.; Gordon, E. Explicit identification and implicit recognition of facial emotions: I. Age effects in males and femals across 10 decades. *J. Clin. Exp. Neuropsychol.* **2009**, *31*, 257–277. [CrossRef]
14. Palermo, R.; Coltheart, M. Photographs of facial expression: Accuracy, response times, and ratings of in-tensity. *Behav. Res. Methods Instrum. Comput.* **2004**, *36*, 634–638. [CrossRef] [PubMed]
15. Hampson, E.; von Anders, S.M.; Mullin, L.I. A female advantage in the recognition of emotional facial ex-pressions: Test of an evolutionary hypothesis. *Evol. Hum. Behav.* **2006**, *27*, 401–416. [CrossRef]
16. Ruffman, T.; Henry, J.D.; Livingstone, V.; Phillips, L.H. A meta-analytic review of emotion recognition and aging: Implications for neuropsychological models of aging. *Neurosci. Behav. Rev.* **2008**, *4*, 863–881. [CrossRef] [PubMed]
17. Von Piekartz, H.; Mohr, G. Reduction of head and face pain by challenging lateralization and basic emotions: A proposal for future assessment and rehabilitation strategies. *J. Man. Manip. Ther.* **2014**, *22*, 24–35. [CrossRef]
18. Lindquist, K.A. Emotions emerge from more basic psychological ingredients: A modern psychological constructionist model. *Emot. Rev.* **2013**, *5*, 356–368. [CrossRef]
19. Palermo-Gallagher, N.; Amunts, K. A short review on emotion processing: A lateralized network o neuronal networks. *Brain Struct. Funct.* **2022**, *227*, 673–684. [CrossRef]
20. Gianotti, G. A historical review of investigations on laterality of emotions in the human brain. *J. Hist. Neurosci.* **2019**, *28*, 23–41. [CrossRef]
21. Mohr, G.; Konnerth, V.; von Piekartz, H.J.M. Lateralitätserkennung und (emotionale) Expressionen des Gesichts—Beurteilung und Behandlung. In *Kiefer, Gesichts-und Zervikalregion*; Thieme: Stuttgart, Germany, 2015; pp. 494–512.
22. Neal, D.T.; Chartrand, T.L. Embodied Emotion Perception: Amplifying and Dampening Facial Feedback modulates Emotion Perception Accuracy. *Soc. Psychol. Personal. Sci.* **2011**, *2*, 673–678. [CrossRef]
23. Goldman, A.I.; Sripada, C.S. Simulationist models of face-based emotion recognition. *Cognition* **2005**, *94*, 193–213. [CrossRef]
24. Bartolome, G. Grundlagen der Funktionellen Dysphagietherapie (FDT): Restituierende Therapieverfahren. In *Schluckstörungen: Diagnostik und Rehabilitation*; Urban & Fischer: München, Germany, 2010; pp. 245–370.
25. Neely, J.G. Central Causes of Facial Paralysis. In *The Facial Nerve*; Thieme: New York, NY, USA, 2014; pp. 129–136.
26. Klingner, C.M.; Witte, O.W. Central Facial Palsy. In *Facial Nerve Disorders and Diseases: Diagnosis and Management*; Thieme: Stuttgart, Germany, 2016; pp. 358–369.
27. Konnerth, V.; Mohr, G.; von Piekartz, H. Fähigkeit von Patienten mit einer peripheren Fazialisparese zur Erkennung von Emotionen—Eine Pilotstudie. *Rehabilitation* **2016**, *55*, 19–25. [CrossRef]
28. Storbeck, F.; Schlegelmilch, K.; Streitberger, K.-J.; Sommer, W.; Ploner, C.J. Delayed recognition of emotional facial expressions in Bell's palsy. *Cortex* **2019**, *120*, 524–531. [CrossRef]
29. Korb, S.; Wood, A.; Banks, C.A.; Agoulnik, D.; Hadlock, T.A.; Niedenthal, P.M. Asymmetry of Facial Mimicry and Emotion Perception in Patients With Unilateral Facial Paralysis. *JAMA Facial Plast. Surg.* **2016**, *18*, 222–227. [CrossRef] [PubMed]
30. Kim, M.J.; Neta, M.; Davis, F.C.; Ruberry, E.J.; Dinescu, D.; Heatherton, T.F.; Stotland, M.A.; Whalen, P.J. Botulinum toxin-induced facial muscle paralysis affects amygdala responses to the perception of emotional expressions: Preliminary findings from an A-B-A design. *Biol. Mood Anxiety Disord.* **2014**, *4*, 1–8. [CrossRef] [PubMed]
31. Strack, F.; Martin, L.L.; Stepper, S. Inhibiting and facilitating conditions of the human smile: A nonobtrusive test of the facial feedback hypothesis. *J. Personal. Soc. Psychol.* **1988**, *54*, 768–777. [CrossRef]
32. Havas, D.A.; Glenberg, A.M.; Gutwoski, K.A.; Lucarelli, M.J.; Davidson, R.J. Cosmetic Use of Botulinum Toxin-A Affects. *Psychol. Sci.* **2010**, *21*, 895–900. [CrossRef]
33. Niedenthal, P.M.; Brauer, M.; Halberstadt, J.B.; Innes-Ker, A.H. When did her smile drop? Facial mimicry and the influences of emotional state on the detection of change in emotional expression. *Cogn. Emot.* **2001**, *15*, 853–864. [CrossRef]
34. Keillor, J.M.; Barrett, A.M.; Crucian, G.P.; Kortenkamp, S.; Heilman, K.M. Emotional experience and perception in the absence of facial feedback. *J. Int. Neuropsychol. Soc.* **2002**, *8*, 130–135. [CrossRef]
35. Bogart, K.R.; Matsumoto, D. Facial mimicry is not necessary to recognize emotion: Facial expression recognition by people with Moebius syndrome. *Soc. Neurosci.* **2010**, *5*, 241–251. [CrossRef]
36. Calder, A.J.; Keane, J.; Cole, J.; Campbell, R.; Young, A.W. Facial Expression Recognition by People with Möbius Syndrome. *Cogn. Neuropsychol.* **2000**, *17*, 73–87. [CrossRef]
37. Kuriakose, D.; Xiao, Z. Pathophysiology and Treatment of Stroke: Present Status und Future Perspectives. *Int. J. Mol. Sci.* **2020**, *21*, 7609. [CrossRef]
38. Armstrong, M.J.; Okun, M.S. Diagnosis and Treatment of Parkinson Disease: A Review. *Jama* **2020**, *323*, 548–560. [CrossRef] [PubMed]

39. Finkensieper, M.; Volk, G.F.; Guntinas-Lichius, O. Erkrankungen des Nervus facialis. *Laryngo-Rhino-Otologie* **2012**, *91*, 121–142. [CrossRef] [PubMed]
40. Bologna, M.; Fabbrini, G.; Marsili, L.; Defazio, G.; Thompson, P.D.; Berardelli, A. Facial bradynkinesia. *J. Neurol. Neurosurg. Psychiatry* **2013**, *84*, 681–685. [CrossRef] [PubMed]
41. Bologna, M.; Berardelli, I.; Paprella, G.; Marsili, L.; Ricciardi, L.; Fabbrini, G.; Berardelli, A. Altered Kinematics of Facial Emotion Expression and Emotion Recognition Deficits Are Unrelated in Parkinson's Disease. *Front. Neurol.* **2016**, *7*, 230. [CrossRef] [PubMed]
42. Marsili, L.; Agostino, R.; Bologna, M.; Belvisi, D.; Palma, A.; Fabbrini, G.; Berardelli, A. Bradykinesia of psed smiling and voluntary movement of the lower face in Parkinson's disease. *Parkinsonism Relat. Disord.* **2014**, *20*, 370–375. [CrossRef]
43. Yuvaraj, R.; Murugappan, M.; Norlinah, M.I.; Sundaraj, K.; Khairiyah, M. Review of Emotion Recognition in Stroke Patients. *Dement. Cogn. Disord.* **2013**, *36*, 179–196. [CrossRef]
44. Vaughan, A.; Copley, A.; Miles, A. Physical rehabilitation of central facial palsy: A survey of current multi-disciplinary practice. *Int. J. Speech-Lang. Pathol.* **2021**, 1–10. [CrossRef]
45. Belin, P.; Fillion-Bilodeau, S.; Gosselin, F. The Montreal Affective Voices: A validated set of nonverbal affect bursts for research on auditory affective processing. *Behav. Res. Methods* **2008**, *40*, 531–539. [CrossRef]
46. Herzer, S.; Maigler, A. Eine Revision der Referenzwerte der sechs Basisemotionen des CRAFTA Face-Mirroring Programms. In *Eine Querschnittstudie*; Hochschule Osnabrück: Osnabrück, Germany, 2016.
47. CRAFTA Cranio Facial Therapy Academy. Operating Guidelines CRAFTA Facemirroring Assessment and Treatment. Available online: https://www.myfacetraining.com/downloads/CRAFTA%20Operating%20Guidelines.pdf (accessed on 28 January 2019).
48. Von Piekartz, H.; Wallwork, S.B.; Mohr, G.; Butler, D.S.; Moseley, G.L. People with chronic facial pain per-form worse than controls at a facial emotion recognition task, but it is not all about the emotion. *J. Oral Rehabil.* **2015**, *42*, 243–250. [CrossRef]
49. Myfacetraining. Available online: https://www.myfacetraining.com/ (accessed on 27 August 2019).
50. Peirce, J.W.; MacAskill, M.R. *Building Experiments in PsychoPy*; Sage: London, UK, 2018.
51. Coulson, S.E.; O'Dwyer, N.J.; Adams, R.D.; Croxson, G.R. Expression of Emotion and Quality of Life After Facial Nerve Paralysis. *Otol. Neurol.* **2004**, *25*, 1014–1019. [CrossRef]
52. Ross, B.G.; Fradet, G.; Nedzelski, J.M. Development of a sensitive clinical facial grading system. *Otolaryngol. Head Neck Surg.* **1996**, *114*, 380–386. [CrossRef]
53. Neumann, T.; Lorenz, A.; Volk, G.F.; Hamzei, F.; Schulz, S.; Guntinas-Lichius, O. Validierung einer Deutschen Version des Sunnybrook Facial Grading Systems. *Laryngo-Rhino-Otologie* **2017**, *96*, 168–174. [CrossRef] [PubMed]
54. Guntinas-Lichius, O.; Finkensieper, M. Grading. In *Facial Nerve Disorders and Diseases: Diagnosis and Management*; Thieme: Stuttgart, Germany, 2016; pp. 94–111.
55. Fattah, A.; Gurusinghe, A.; Gavilan, J.; Hadlock, T.; Markus, J.; Marres, H.; Nduka, C.; Slattery, W.; Snyder-Warwick, A. Facial Nerve Grading Instruments: Systematic Review of the Literature and Suggestion for Uniformity. *Plast. Reconstr. Surg.* **2015**, *135*, 569–579. [CrossRef] [PubMed]
56. Akulov, M.A.; Orlova, A.S.; Usachev, D.J.; Shimansky, V.N.; Tanjashin, S.V.; Khatkova, S.E.; Yunosha-Shanyavskaya, A.V. IncobotulinumtoxinA treatment of facial nerve palsy after neurosurgery. *J. Neurol. Sci.* **2017**, *381*, 130–134. [CrossRef]
57. Beurskens, C.H.; Heymans, P.G. Mime therapy improves facial symmetry in people with long-term facial nerve paresis: A randomised controlled trail. *Aust. J. Physiother.* **2006**, *52*, 177–183. [CrossRef]
58. Goo, B.; Jeong, S.M.; Kim, J.U.; Park, Y.C.; Seo, B.K.; Baek, Y.H.; Yook, T.H.; Nam, S.S. Clinical efficacy and safety of thread-embedding acupuncture for treatment of the sequelae of Bell's palsy: A protocol for a patient-assessor blinded, randomized, controlled, parallel clinical trial. *Medicine* **2019**, *98*, e14508. [CrossRef]
59. Kim, J.; Choi, J.Y. The effect of subthreshold continuous electrical stimulation on the facial function of patients with Bell's palsy. *Acta Oto-Laryngol.* **2016**, *136*, 100–105. [CrossRef]
60. Kuttenreich, A.-M.; Rethfeldt, W.S.; von Piekartz, H. Autobiografische Erinnerungen bei Behandlung zentraler Fazialisparesen. *Forum Logopädie* **2018**, *32*, 6–13.
61. Kwon, H.-J.; Choi, J.-Y.; Lee, M.S.; Kim, Y.-S.; Shin, B.-C.; Kim, J.-I. Acupuncture for the sequelae of Bell's palsy: A randomized controlled trial. *Trails* **2015**, *16*, 246–253. [CrossRef]
62. Ton, G.; Lee, L.W.; Ng, H.P.; Liao, H.Y.; Chen, Y.H.; Tu, C.H.; Tseng, C.H.; Ho, W.C.; Lee, Y.C. Efficacy of laser acupuncture for patients with chronic Bell's palsy: A study protocol for a randomized, double-blind, sham-controlled pilot trial. *Medicine* **2019**, *98*, e15120. [CrossRef]
63. Cambridge Dictionary. Quick and Dirty. 2020. Available online: https://dictionary.cambridge.org/de/worterbuch/englisch/quick-and-dirty (accessed on 9 September 2020).
64. Deutsche Gesellschaft für Allgemeinmedizin und Familienmedizin (DEGAM). DEGAM-Leitlinie Nr. 8 Schlaganfall. 2012. Available online: https://www.awmf.org/uploads/tx_szleitlinien/053-011l_S3_Schlaganfall_2012-abgelaufen.pdf (accessed on 23 June 2018).
65. Sánchez-Lozano, E.; Lopez-Otero, P.; Docio-Fernandez, L.; Argones-Rúa, E.; Alba-Castro, J.L. Audiovisual Three-Level Fusion for Continuous Estimation of Russell's emotion Circumplex. In Proceedings of the 3rd ACM International Workshop on Audio/Visual Emotion Challenge, Barcelona, Spain, 21 October 2013; pp. 31–40.

66. Bundesarbeitsgemeinschaft für Rehabilitation. Arbeitshilfe für die Rehabilitation von Schlaganfallpatienten. 1998. Available online: https://www.bar-frankfurt.de/service/publikationen/produktdetails/produkt/65.html (accessed on 23 September 2019).
67. World Health Organization (WHO). Internationale Klassifikation der Funktionsfähigkeit, Behinderung und Gesundheit (ICF). 2005. Available online: https://www.dimdi.de/dynamic/de/klassifikationen/downloads/?dir=icf (accessed on 18 September 2019).
68. Coles, N.A.; Larsen, J.T.; Lench, H.C. A Meta-Analysis of the Facial Feedback Literature: Effects of Facial Feedback on Emotion Experience Are Small and Variable. *Psychol. Bull.* **2019**, *145*, 610–651. [CrossRef] [PubMed]
69. Dobel, C.; Miltner, W.H.R.; Witte, O.W.; Volk, G.F.; Guntinas-Lichius, O. Emotionale Auswirkung einer Fazialisparese. *Laryngo-Rhino-Otologie* **2013**, *92*, 9–23. [PubMed]
70. Taylor, G.J.; Bagby, R.M. An overview of the alexithymia construct. In *The Handbook of Emotional Intelligence: Theory, Development, Assessment, and Application at Home, School, and in the Workplace*; Jossey-Bass: San Francisco, CA, USA, 2000; pp. 40–67.
71. Beushausen, U.; Grötzbach, H. *Evidenzbasierte Sprachtherapie: Grundlagen und Praxis*; Elsevier: München, Germany, 2011.
72. Dollaghan, C. *The Handbook for Evidence-Based Practice in Communication Disorders*; Paul H. Books: Baltimore, MD, USA, 2007.
73. Gilden, D.H. Clinical Practice: Bell's Palsy. *N. Engl. J. Med.* **2004**, *351*, 1323–1331. [CrossRef] [PubMed]
74. Hildebrandt, A.; Sommer, W.; Schacht, A.; Wilhelm, O. Perceiving and remembering emotional facial ex-pressions—A basis facet of emotional intelligence. *Intelligence* **2015**, *50*, 52–67. [CrossRef]
75. Olderbak, S.; Semmler, M.; Doebler, P. Four-branch model of ability emotion intelligence with fluid and crystallized intelligence: A meta-analysis of relations. *Emot. Rev.* **2019**, *11*, 166–183. [CrossRef]
76. Schlegel, K.; Palese, T.; Mast, M.S.; Rammsayer, T.H.; Hall, J.A.; Murphy, N.A. A meta-analysis of the relationship between emotion recognition ability and intelligence. *Cogn. Emot.* **2020**, *2*, 329–351. [CrossRef]
77. Ricciardi, L.; Visco-Comandini, F.; Erro, R.; Morgante, F.; Volpe, D.; Kilner, J.; Edwards, M.J.; Bologna, M. Emotional facedness in Parkinson's disease. *J. Neural Transm.* **2018**, *125*, 1819–1827. [CrossRef]
78. Rosenberg, H.; McDonald, S.; Rosenberg, J.; Westbrook, R.F. Measuring emotion perception following traumatic brain injury: The Complex Audio Visual Emotion Assessment Task (CAVEAT). *Neuropsychol. Rehabil.* **2019**, *29*, 232–250. [CrossRef]
79. House, J.W.; Brackmann, D.E. Facial nerve grading system. *Otolaryngol.-Head Neck Surg.* **1985**, *93*, 146–147. [CrossRef]
80. Online Psychology Research. Montreal Affective Voices. Available online: https://experiments.psy.gla.ac.uk//index.php (accessed on 11 June 2018).
81. Paquette, S.; Peretz, I.; Belin, P. The "Musical Emotional Bursts": A validated set of musical affect bursts to investigate auditory affective processing. *Front. Psychol.* **2013**, *4*, 509. [CrossRef]
82. Miller, M.Q.; Hadlock, T.A.; Fortier, E.; Guarin, D.L. The Auto-eFACE: Machine Learning-Enhanced Program Yields Automated Facial Palsy Assessment Tool. *Plast. Reconstr. Surg.* **2021**, *147*, 467–474. [CrossRef] [PubMed]

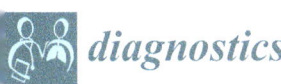

Article

Intratemporal Facial Nerve Schwannomas: A Review of 45 Cases in A Single Center

Tsubasa Kitama [1], Makoto Hosoya [1], Masaru Noguchi [1], Takanori Nishiyama [1], Takeshi Wakabayashi [1], Marie N. Shimanuki [1], Masaki Yazawa [2], Yasuhiro Inoue [1], Jin Kanzaki [1], Kaoru Ogawa [1] and Naoki Oishi [1,*]

[1] Department of Otorhinolaryngology-Head and Neck Surgery, Keio University School of Medicine, 35 Shinanomachi, Shinjuku-ku, Tokyo 160-8582, Japan; tsubasa.kitama@gmail.com (T.K.); mhosoya1985@gmail.com (M.H.); masaru_n0613@yahoo.co.jp (M.N.); tnmailster@gmail.com (T.N.); t12wakabayashi@yahoo.co.jp (T.W.); nukimari@gmail.com (M.N.S.); yas712hachiman@gmail.com (Y.I.); kanj1937@yahoo.co.jp (J.K.); ogawak@a5.keio.jp (K.O.)

[2] Department of Plastic Surgery, Keio University School of Medicine, 35 Shinanomachi, Shinjuku-ku, Tokyo 160-8582, Japan; yazawa@a7.keio.jp

* Correspondence: oishin@keio.jp; Tel.: +81-3-3353-1211

Abstract: There are no established indications for facial nerve schwannoma treatment, including surgery, radiation and follow-up observation, and it is difficult to determine treatment policy uniformly. The treatment policy was examined from each treatment course. Data of patients with facial nerve schwannomas at our hospital from 1987 to 2018 were retrospectively examined. Their age, sex, clinical symptoms, tumor localization, treatment policies and outcomes were reviewed. In total, 22 patients underwent surgery and 1 patient underwent radiotherapy; 22 patients were followed up without treatment. After total resection, there were no tumor recurrences, and most patients had grade 3 or 4 postoperative facial paralysis. After subtotal resection, tumor regrowth was observed in four patients and reoperation was required in two patients. Facial nerve function was maintained in four patients and was decreased in two patients. During follow-up, six patients showed tumor growth. Only one patient had worsening facial nerve paralysis; four patients underwent facial nerve decompression owing to facial nerve paralysis during follow-up. If the tumor compresses the brain or it is prone to growth, surgery may be indicated, and when the preoperative facial nerve function is grade ≤ 3, consideration should be given to preserving facial nerve function and subtotal resection should be indicated. If the preoperative facial nerve function is grade ≥ 3, total resection with nerve grafting is an option to prevent regrowth. If there is no brain compression or tumor growth, the follow-up is a good indication, and decompression should be considered in facial nerve paralysis cases.

Keywords: facial nerve schwannomas; facial nerve palsy; temporal bone

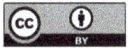

1. Introduction

Facial nerve schwannoma is the most frequent tumor derived from the facial nerve [1]. It is benign and commonly grows slowly. It can occur at any location in the facial nerve, from near the brainstem to outside the temporal bone. The most common site of occurrence is in the temporal bone facial nerve canal, followed by the cerebellar pons, inner ear canal and parotid gland [2]. Previous studies have found sporadic facial nerve schwannoma in <1% of the temporal bone [3], but in clinical practice, it is often found during the close investigation of facial nerve paralysis. Facial nerve schwannoma may cause several other symptoms such as hearing loss, tinnitus, vertigo, cephalalgia and otalgia. When it increases and compresses the brain, it may cause neurological symptoms and signs such as paralysis and trigeminal neuralgia [4].

Although facial nerve schwannoma treatment mainly includes surgical intervention, radiation and follow-up observation, there are no established criteria for treatment selection [5]. Follow-up observation is an option for patients without facial paralysis and tumor growth. Total resection was the main surgical intervention until the 90s, but it has been recently limited to the tumors with progressive palsy or tumors that compress the brainstem, temporal lobe or cerebellum. Total resection requires nerve resection and reconstruction [2]. Subtotal resection has been a treatment option after the 2000s. Some reviews have shown that this operation enables nerve preservation by limiting the procedure to tumor debulking [6].

There are insufficient studies on the long-term course after subtotal resection. Facial nerve decompression can be performed when the tumor causes facial nerve paralysis during observation [7,8]. Some studies have reported the validity of radiation therapy, including gamma knife treatment. During the follow-up period of approximately 5 years, approximately 30% of the target cases require postoperative irradiation. The rate of good control is approximately 90%, and the facial nerve function improvement rate is 20%. In contrast, facial nerve function deterioration rates of 10–20% have been reported [9,10]. Most studies have evaluated tumors near the cistern, and there are limited studies on tumors in the temporal bone.

In facial schwannoma treatment, facial nerve function preservation has become increasingly important. Tumor regrowth after treatment should also be avoided as much as possible. There are many cases in which no increase or worsening of facial nerve paralysis is observed without treatment. Taken together, there are no established criteria regarding which case should be treated and which treatment option should be chosen. This study aimed to investigate the outcome of each treatment based on the largest number of cases in Japan to consider indications for each treatment.

2. Materials and Methods

The data of patients who were treated or observed at the Department of Otorhinolaryngology at Keio University Hospital from 1987 to 2018 (32 years) were retrospectively examined. This survey was approved by the Institutional Review Board of Keio University (Ethics Numbers 20140242, 20200033).

Their age, sex, clinical symptoms, tumor localization and treatment policies were reviewed. Tumor localization was classified into the cerebellopontine angle (CPA), internal auditory canal (IAC), geniculate ganglion (GG), horizontal portion of the facial nerve (H), vertical portion of the facial nerve (V) and parotid gland (PA).

3. Results

In total, 45 patients visited our outpatient department during the study period. There were 22 men and 23 women with a mean age of 43.9 years (13–74 years). Among the 23 patients with facial nerve paralysis, 16 had gradually advanced facial nerve paralysis, 4 had recurrent facial nerve paralysis and 3 had sudden-onset facial nerve paralysis. Among the 26 patients with hearing loss, 23 had conductive hearing loss, 7 had tinnitus, 4 had ear fullness and 2 had dizziness; 7 other patients had ear canal mass, 2 had otorrhea and 2 had parotid gland mass. Figure 1 shows the location of the tumor. Most tumors straddled >1 segment.

Regarding the location of the tumor, five tumors straddled the CPA, IAC and GG; five straddled the CPA, ICA, GG, H and V; two straddled the IAC and GG; two straddled the IAC, GG and H; two straddled the IAC, GG, H and V; six straddled the GG; four straddled the GG and H; three straddled the GG, H and V; two straddled the GG, H, V and Pa, three straddled the H; six straddled the H and V; one straddled the H, V and Pa; five straddled the V; and two straddled the V and PA. Among the 10 tumors extending to the CPA, 7 caused facial nerve paralysis. Among the 16 tumors extending to the IAC, 9 caused facial nerve paralysis. Among the 30 tumors extending to the GG, 16 caused facial nerve paralysis. Among the 26 tumors extending to the H, 11 caused facial nerve paralysis. Among the 25 tumors extending to the V, 13 caused facial nerve paralysis. Among the five tumors extending to the PA, one caused facial nerve paralysis.

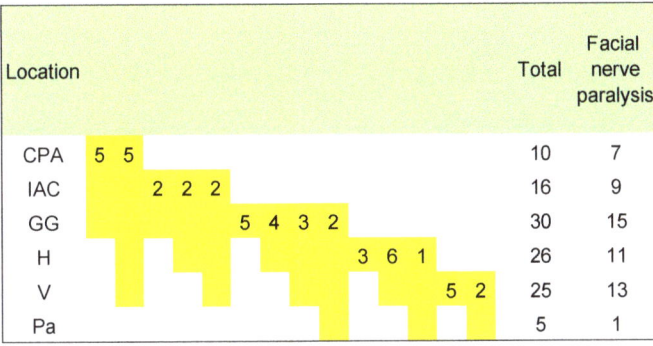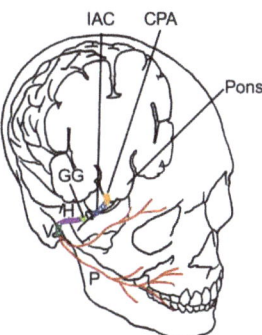

Figure 1. Tumor location and facial nerve function. CPA: cerebellopontine angle, IAC: internal auditory canal, GG: geniculate ganglion, H: horizontal portion of the facial nerve, V: vertical portion of the facial nerve, PA: parotid gland.

The treatment policy was also examined and 22 patients eventually underwent operation; 16 underwent total resection and 6 underwent subtotal resection. One patient underwent radiotherapy and 22 patients were followed up without treatment; 4 of them underwent facial nerve decompression. Table 1 shows the features of patients treated with each treatment policy and Table 2 shows the outcomes of each treatment policy.

Table 1. Features of patients with each treatment policy.

		Total Resection (n = 16)	Subtotal Resection (n = 6)	Follow-up (n = 22)
	Age (Mean ± Standard Deviation)	48.1 ± 16.7	40.2 ± 12.5	44.1 ± 17.4
Sex	Male	8	3	10
	Female	8	3	12
Facial nerve paralysis	Grade 1, 2	9	5	15
	Grade 3, 4	4	1	5
	Grade 5, 6	3	0	2

This table shows the patients' features who underwent the following treatment: total resection, subtotal resection and follow-up. There is no tendency for age or sex in each treatment group, but it can be seen that there are many mild cases of facial nerve paralysis in the follow-up group and relatively many severe cases in the total resection group.

This table shows the outcomes of those who underwent the following treatment: total resection, subtotal resection and follow-up. Most facial nerve paralysis after total excision was grade 3 or 4 in the total-resection group. Many patients had preserved facial nerve function in the subtotal-resection group and the follow-up group. Tumors regrew in six patients during the observation. Among them, two patients underwent total resection, one underwent subtotal resection, two received radiation therapy and one was followed up.

The average age of patients who underwent total resection was 48.1 years (13–68 years), and there were eight men and eight women. Regarding preoperative facial nerve condition, nine patients were House–Brackmann grade [11] 1 and 2, four were grade 3 and 4, and three were grade 5. The amputated facial nerve was reconstructed with the hypoglossal nerve in eight cases and reconstructed with the nerve grafts of the auricular nerve or sural nerve in seven cases. There were no tumor recurrences after surgery. In most cases, postoperative facial paralysis was grade 3 or 4. Exceptionally, in three cases, the tumor derived from the large pyramidal nerve and the intermediate nerve was grade 1 or 2.

Table 2. Outcomes of each treatment policy.

	Total Resection (n = 16)	Subtotal Resection (n = 6)	Follow-up (n = 22)
HB grade at diagnosis			
1	5	4	13
2	4	1	2
3	3	1	2
4	1	0	3
5	3	0	2
6	0	0	0
HB grade at last follow-up			
1	1	3	14
2	2	2	3
3	5	1	2
4	5	0	2
5	3	0	1
6	0	0	0
Change in HB grade			
Same or improved	7	4	20
Worse	9	2	2
Cases in which the treament policy was changed during follow-up			
total resection			2
subtotal resection			1
radiation therapy			2

The average age of patients who underwent subtotal resection was 40.2 years (17–54 years), and regarding sex there were three males and three females. Regarding the preoperative facial nerve condition, four, one, one, and zero patients were classified as having House–Brackmann grades 1, 2, 3, and ≥4, respectively. The operation was performed via the middle fossa or transmastoid approach, and the tumor was removed using a nerve integrity monitor as much as possible. Tumor regrowth was noted in four patients after operation: two were completely resected and two were followed up. Postoperative facial nerve paralysis was grade 1 in three patients, grade 2 in two patients and grade 3 in one patient. In three patients, conductive hearing loss was observed before surgery; therefore, type IV reconstruction was performed, which improved hearing.

The average age of the initially followed-up patients was 44.1 years (16–74 years), and there were 10 men and 12 women. Regarding the facial nerve condition at the first visit, 13, 2, 2, 3, and 2 patients were classified as having grades 1, 2, 3, 4, and 5, respectively. Tumors grew in six patients during the observation. Among them, four patients showed tumor growth in the CPA, of which two patients underwent total excision, one underwent radiation therapy and one was followed up. Further, two patients showed tumor growth in the GG: one patient underwent debulking surgery and the other patient received radiation therapy. Tumors in the H or V showed little growth. During observation, 2 patients had worsening facial nerve paralysis, and the remaining 20 had preserved facial nerve function.

Four patients underwent facial nerve decompression. Their average age was 30.8 years (24–40 years), and there were two men and two women. Regarding the facial nerve condition at the first visit, one, one, one, and one patient was classified as having grades 1, 3, 4, and 5, respectively. The duration of paralysis was <3 weeks in two patients, who were classified as having grades 3 and 5; approximately 2 months in one patient, who was classified as having grade 4; and >1 year (chronic) in the remaining one patient, who was classified as having grade 2. Only one patient with facial nerve paralysis recovered after operation (from grade 5 to grade 1). In the recovered patient, the tumor was in the vertical portion, and the preoperative electroneurography value was 0%. The operation was performed 3 weeks after the onset.

4. Discussion

Treatment for facial schwannoma has changed over time, and because it is a rare tumor, there are various debates regarding the treatment options [12]. Tumors do not often regrow even after subtotal resection, and facial nerve paralysis greatly impairs the quality of life. Malignant tumor transformation is extremely rare, and diagnostic imaging of the tumor by CT and MRI becomes accurate. There is a tendency to prioritize the preservation of facial nerve function over total tumor removal. In this study, the data of patients who were followed up or treated at our department were retrospectively considered to examine treatment strategies.

In this study, 22 patients were initially followed up. In all patients, the tumors did not compress the brain, and most patients had maintained facial nerve function of House–Brackmann grade 1 or 2. In some patients, even if facial nerve paralysis was grade $\geq$ 3, the tumors that did not show a tendency to grow were followed up with periodic imaging. Less than 30% of the tumors grew during follow-up and only one patient had worsened facial nerve function. Preservation of facial nerve function should be prioritized generally, and conservative follow-up is the first choice rather than interventional treatment such as surgery and radiation therapy. If there is no brain compression and no facial nerve paralysis of House–Brackmann grade $\geq$ 3, follow-up should be performed first. Some reports show that the average annual growth of the tumor is approximately 1–2 mm [5], and larger tumors are more likely to cause subsequent growth [13]. Follow-up with careful imaging is essential. If facial nerve paralysis occurs during follow-up, steroids should be administered first. Facial nerve decompression should be considered, especially for intratemporal tumors in an early stage [8]. In this study, among the four patients with decompression, one recovered and the condition of three did not worsen.

Surgery for schwannoma can be divided into total or subtotal resection. In this study, 16 patients underwent total resection. Regarding total resection, there are many cases in which the tumor and nerve are unclearly marginated, and nerve fibers are found almost all around the tumor, especially in the temporal bone. Thus, total excision of the tumor in the temporal bone or brain cistern is not usually able to avoid facial nerve paralysis. Before 2000s, total tumor resection was performed for almost all cases [7,14]. When total resection with nerve grafting is achieved, good long-term tumor control and facial nerve function of House–Brackmann grade 3–4 are expected. In this study, facial nerve function was not preserved after surgery in all patients without tumor recurrence except cases with tumors originated from the large pyramidal nerve or the intermediate nerve, and most facial nerve paralysis after total excision was grade 3 or 4. Liu et al. reported that facial nerve paralysis after total resection was almost House–Brackmann grade 3 [15]. If the preoperative House–Brackmann grade is $\geq$3, total tumor resection and nerve transplant reconstruction are indicated. Similar opinions have been expressed in previous literature [16,17]. The facial nerve function after reconstruction improves as the period of facial nerve paralysis before surgery becomes shorter. Surgery should be considered as soon as possible once facial nerve paralysis has progressed to grade 3 or 4 [2,18].

Although there are insufficient studies on the long-term course after subtotal resection, some studies have shown good nerve-sparing rates after resection for tumors from the cerebellar pontine corner to the inner ear canal [6,19]. In six patients included in this study, four achieved preservation of the facial nerve function. Deterioration of the facial nerve function was observed in two patients but it was very mild. Further, four of six (66.7%) patients had tumor regrowth, and two patients finally required reoperation. Previous literature also reported a recurrence rate of 26.7% [20], and there is a risk of regrowth with subtotal resection. Previously, nerve monitoring using a nerve integrity monitor was used. Recently, continuous monitoring of facial nerves using the facial nerve root exit-zone-elicited compound muscle action potential has become possible [21–23], and there is a possibility that the nerve preservation rate can be further increased in the future. It may be an effective option for growing tumors if patients are relatively young and have good facial nerve function. There is also a treatment algorithm that positions subtotal resection as a treatment option for intracranial tumors measuring >3 cm that maintain good facial nerve function [24].

Regarding the surgical method, various surgical methods, such as the suboccipital craniotomy approach, the middle cranial fossa approach, the translabyrinthine approach, the approach that combines the middle cranial fossa with transmastoid, the transmastoid approach, excision according to the parotid tumor and temporal bone surgery with parotid gland surgery, are used depending on the location of the tumor, degree of residual hearing and experience of the operator [2]. It is necessary to be familiar with various approaches in each area of temporal bone surgery, head and neck surgery, neurosurgery and plastic surgery. Surgical treatment in an experienced facility that can provide team medical care by multiple departments is desirable.

For parotid gland tumors, it is necessary to consider the natural course, as facial nerve paralysis rarely occurs during the follow-up period. A treatment algorithm has been proposed according to whether the tumor extends intratemporally [25]. In the case of intratemporal extension, follow-up after decompression is recommended. In the case without intratemporal extension and if the tumor can be detached from the nerve or if the tumor occurs in a peripheral branch rather than the main trunk, total resection with nerve grafting is recommended. If detachment from the nerve is difficult, follow-up is recommended.

Radiation therapy is a good treatment option for patients with a tendency for tumor growth but with good facial nerve function, such as House–Brackmann grade 1–3 [26]. The treatment outcomes for tumors located more centrally from the geniculate ganglion have been reported. The treatment outcomes for tumors in the temporal bone are unknown [9]. Radiation therapy has not been confirmed to be effective for facial nerve schwannoma of the temporal bone and is not an active indication at the moment.

Facial nerve paralysis is the most important symptom of facial nerve schwannoma, which especially affects quality of life, and it has been examined from the same viewpoint in the past [2,7,8,27]. Thus, the treatment indication was examined from facial nerve paralysis and tumor growth mainly in this study. Facial nerve schwannoma also causes hearing loss, dysgeusia and ocular symptoms, so it may be necessary to consider the treatment policy from such a viewpoint in addition.

5. Conclusions

Figure 2 shows the treatment strategies for intratemporal facial nerve schwannoma. If the tumor compresses the brain or if the tumor is prone to growth, surgery may be indicated, and when the preoperative facial nerve function is grade ≤ 3, consideration should be given to preserving facial nerve function, and subtotal resection should be indicated. If it is grade ≥ 3, total resection with nerve grafting is an option to prevent regrowth. If there is no brain compression or tumor growth, follow-up is a good indication, and when facial paralysis appears, decompression should be considered.

Treatment strategies for intratemporal facial nerve schwannoma are first divided according to whether the tumor is compressing the brain. If the brain is compressed, or if tumor is prone to grow, surgical treatment is indicated. If the facial nerve paralysis is H-B grade 1–3, subtotal resection is required, and if H-B grade is 3–6, total resection is required. If no compression of the brain and no tumor growth is observed, patients should be followed up. If acute facial paralysis develops during follow-up, decompression should be considered.

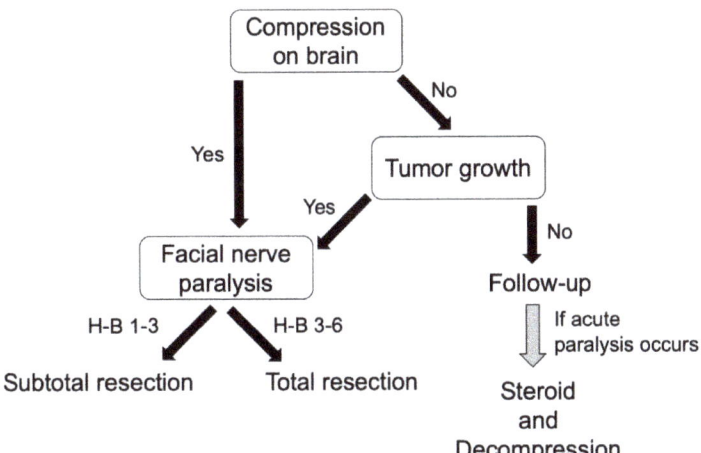

Figure 2. Treatment policies for intratemporal facial nerve schwannoma.

Author Contributions: Conceptualization, T.K., M.H. and N.O.; methodology, N.O.; formal analysis, T.K.; investigation, T.K., M.H., T.N., T.W., M.N.S., M.Y., Y.I. and N.O.; resources, M.N., Y.I., J.K., K.O. and N.O.; data curation, T.K.; writing—original draft preparation, T.K.; writing—review and editing, M.H. and N.O.; visualization, T.K.; supervision, N.O.; project administration, N.O. All authors have read and agreed to the published version of the manuscript.

Funding: This research received no external funding.

Institutional Review Board Statement: The study was conducted in accordance with the Declaration of Helsinki, and approved by the Institutional Review Board of Keio University (Ethics Numbers 20200033 27 April 2020, and 20140242 27 October 2014)".

Informed Consent Statement: Details of this clinical research study were displayed in a consultation room and in our website (https://ent-otol.med.keio.ac.jp/, accessed on 23 August 2021). According to the Japan Ethical Guidelines for Medical and Health Research Involving Human Subjects, obtaining informed consent for observational studies is not required. We notified the research subjects, or made public, information concerning the research, including the purpose of collecting and using the research information. We also informed the participants that they could refuse participation at any time or could request that their data be removed from the study after commencement.

Data Availability Statement: The datasets generated and analyzed during the current study are available from the corresponding author on reasonable request.

Acknowledgments: We acknowledge the support of the Department of Otorhinolaryngology, Keio University Hospital.

Conflicts of Interest: The authors declare no conflict of interest.

References

1. McRackan, T.R.; Wilkinson, E.P.; Rivas, A. Primary Tumors of the Facial Nerve. *Otolaryngol. Clin. N. Am.* **2015**, *48*, 491–500. [CrossRef] [PubMed]
2. McMonagle, B.; Al-Sanosi, A.; Croxson, G.R.; A Fagan, P. Facial schwannoma: Results of a large case series and review. *J. Laryngol. Otol.* **2008**, *122*, 1139–1150. [CrossRef] [PubMed]
3. Saito, H.; Baxter, A. Undiagnosed intratemporal facial nerve neurilemomas. *Arch. Otolaryngol.* **1972**, *95*, 415–419. [CrossRef] [PubMed]
4. Sterkers, O.; Viala, P.; Rivière, F.; Sterkers, J.M. Neurinoma of the intratemporal facial nerve. Anatomo-clinical classification of 12 cases. *Ann. Otolaryngol. Chir. Cervicofac.* **1986**, *103*, 501–508. [PubMed]
5. Perez, R.; Chen, J.M.; Nedzelski, J.M. Intratemporal facial nerve schwannoma: A management dilemma. *Otol. Neurotol.* **2005**, *26*, 121–126. [CrossRef] [PubMed]
6. Mowry, S.; Hansen, M.; Gantz, B. Surgical management of internal auditory canal and cerebellopontine angle facial nerve schwannoma. *Otol. Neurotol.* **2012**, *33*, 1071–1076. [CrossRef]

7. Angeli, S.I.; Brackmann, D.E. Is surgical excision of facial nerve schwannomas always indicated? *Otolaryngol. Head Neck Surg.* **1997**, *117*, S144–S147. [CrossRef]
8. Carlson, M.L.; Deep, N.L.; Patel, N.S.; Lundy, L.B.; Tombers, N.M.; Lohse, C.M.; Link, M.J.; Driscoll, C.L. Facial Nerve Schwannomas: Review of 80 Cases Over 25 Years at Mayo Clinic. *Mayo Clin. Proc.* **2016**, *91*, 1563–1576. [CrossRef]
9. Sheehan, J.P.; Kano, H.; Xu, Z.; Chiang, V.; Mathieu, D.; Chao, S.; Akpinar, B.; Lee, J.Y.; Yu, J.B.; Hess, J.; et al. Gamma Knife radiosurgery for facial nerve schwannomas: A multicenter study. *J. Neurosurg.* **2015**, *123*, 387–394. [CrossRef]
10. Hasegawa, T.; Kato, T.; Kida, Y.; Hayashi, M.; Tsugawa, T.; Iwai, Y.; Sato, M.; Okamoto, H.; Kano, T.; Osano, S.; et al. Gamma Knife surgery for patients with facial nerve schwannomas: A multiinstitutional retrospective study in Japan. *J. Neurosurg.* **2016**, *124*, 403–410. [CrossRef]
11. House, J.W. Facial nerve grading systems. *Laryngoscope* **1983**, *93*, 1056–1069. [CrossRef] [PubMed]
12. Cho, Y.S.; Choi, J.E.; Lim, J.H.; Cho, Y.S. Management of facial nerve schwannoma: When is the timing for surgery. *Eur. Arch. Otorhinolaryngol.* **2022**, *279*, 1243–1249. [CrossRef]
13. Yang, W.; Zhao, J.; Han, Y.; Yang, H.; Xing, J.; Zhang, Y.; Wang, Y.; Liu, H. Long-term outcomes of facial nerve schwannomas with favorable facial nerve function: Tumor growth rate is correlated with initial tumor size. *Am. J. Otolaryngol.* **2015**, *36*, 163–165. [CrossRef]
14. Wilkinson, E.P.; Hoa, M.; Slattery, W.H.; Fayad, J.N.; Friedman, R.A.; Schwartz, M.S.; Brackmann, D.E. Evolution in the management of facial nerve schwannoma. *Laryngoscope* **2011**, *121*, 2065–2074. [CrossRef] [PubMed]
15. Liu, R.; Fagan, P. Facial Nerve schwannoma: Surgical excision versus conservative management. *Ann. Otol. Rhinol. Laryngol.* **2001**, *110*, 1025–1029. [CrossRef] [PubMed]
16. Bacciu, A.; Medina, M.; Ben Ammar, M.; D'Orazio, F.; Di Lella, F.; Russo, A.; Magnan, J.; Sanna, M. Intraoperatively diagnosed cerebellopontine angle facial nerve schwannoma: How to deal with it. *Ann. Otol. Rhinol. Laryngol.* **2014**, *123*, 647–653. [CrossRef]
17. Eshraghi, A.A.; Oker, N.; Ocak, E.; Verillaud, B.; Babcock, T.; Camous, D.; Kravietz, A.; Morcos, J.; Herman, P.; Kania, R. Management of Facial Nerve Schwannoma: A Multicenter Study of 50 Cases. *J. Neurol. Surg. B Skull Base* **2019**, *80*, 352–356. [CrossRef]
18. Ozmen, O.A.; Falcioni, M.; Lauda, L.; Sanna, M. Outcomes of facial nerve grafting in 155 cases: Predictive value of history and preoperative function. *Otol. Neurotol.* **2011**, *32*, 1341–1346. [CrossRef]
19. McRackan, T.R.; Rivas, A.; Wanna, G.B.; Yoo, M.J.; Bennett, M.L.; Deitrich, M.S.; Glasscock, M.E.; Haynes, D.S. Facial nerve outcomes in facial nerve schwannomas. *Otol. Neurotol.* **2012**, *33*, 78–82. [CrossRef]
20. Li, Y.; Liu, H.; Cheng, Y. Subtotal resection of facial nerve schwannoma is not safe in the long run. *Acta Otolaryngol.* **2014**, *134*, 433–436. [CrossRef]
21. Hosoya, M.; Oishi, N.; Nishiyama, T.; Noguchi, M.; Kasuya, K.; Suzuki, N.; Miyazaki, H.; Ogawa, K. Preoperative electrophysiological analysis predicts preservation of hearing and facial nerve function following vestibular schwannoma surgery with continuous intraoperative neural monitoring: Clinical outcomes of 22 cases. *Clin. Otolaryngol.* **2019**, *44*, 875–880. [CrossRef] [PubMed]
22. Amano, M.; Kohno, M.; Nagata, O.; Taniguchi, M.; Sora, S.; Sato, H. Intraoperative continuous monitoring of evoked facial nerve electromyograms in acoustic neuroma surgery. *Acta Neurochir.* **2011**, *153*, 1059–1067. [CrossRef] [PubMed]
23. Hosoya, M.; Wakabayashi, T.; Wasano, K.; Nishiyama, T.; Tsuzuki, N.; Oishi, N. Understanding the Molecular Mechanism of Vestibular Schwannoma for Hearing Preservation Surgery: Otologists' Perspective from Bedside to Bench. *Diagnostics* **2022**, *12*, 1044. [CrossRef] [PubMed]
24. Xu, F.; Pan, S.; Alonso, F.; Dekker, S.E.; Bambakidis, N.C. Intracranial Facial Nerve Schwannomas: Current Management and Review of Literature. *World Neurosurg.* **2017**, *100*, 444–449. [CrossRef]
25. Gross, B.C.; Carlson, M.L.; Moore, E.J.; Driscoll, C.L.; Olsen, K.D. The intraparotid facial nerve schwannoma: A diagnostic and management conundrum. *Am. J. Otolaryngol.* **2012**, *33*, 497–504. [CrossRef] [PubMed]
26. Loos, E.; Verhaert, N.; Darrouzet, V.; Godey, B.; Linder, T.; Vincent, C.; Lavieille, J.P.; Schmerber, S.; Lescane, E.; Trabalzini, F.; et al. Intratemporal facial nerve schwannomas: Multicenter experience of 80 cases. *Eur. Arch. Otorhinolaryngol.* **2020**, *277*, 2209–2217. [CrossRef]
27. Quesnel, A.M.; Santos, F. Evaluation and Management of Facial Nerve Schwannoma. *Otolaryngol. Clin. N. Am.* **2018**, *51*, 1179–1192. [CrossRef]

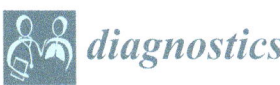

Comment

Comment on Kehrer et al. Using High-Resolution Ultrasound to Assess Post-Facial Paralysis Synkinesis—Machine Settings and Technical Aspects for Facial Surgeons. *Diagnostics* 2022, 12, 1650

Charles Nduka [1], Ruben Yap Kannan [1], Gerd Fabian Volk [2,*] and Orlando Guntinas-Lichius [2]

1. Facial Palsy Unit, Department of Plastic & Reconstructive Surgery, Queen Victoria Hospital, East Grinstead RH19 3DZ, UK
2. Facial-Nerve-Center Jena, Department of Otorhinolaryngology, Center of Rare Diseases Jena, Jena University Hospital, Am Klinikum 1, 07747 Jena, Germany
* Correspondence: fabian.volk@med.uni-jena.de; Tel.: +49-(0)-36419329396

In "Using High-Resolution Ultrasound to Assess Post-Facial Paralysis Synkinesis—Machine Settings and Technical Aspects for Facial Surgeons", Andreas Kehrer et al. present ultrasound (US) device settings for facial muscle examination to be used by facial surgeons to improve their workflow and enhance their image quality [1]. The step-by-step structured working protocol, starting with basic but very important machine settings, should be helpful to conduct more insightful examinations in patients with different kinds of facial palsies.

We strongly encourage the use of facial US not only to capture high-quality US images, but also to quantify these images to acquire metrics related to the various muscles. Indeed, we have previously published detailed Instructions for Sonography of the Mimic Musculature as a part of the book Management of Post-Facial Paralysis Synkinesis [2].

These instructions for sonography of the mimic musculature help sonographers to better understand the complex sonographic cross-sections of the mimic and masticatory musculature and help one to achieve reproducible and quantifiable scans. Because of the special anatomy of the mimic musculature, it is not always easy to differentiate single mimic muscles from the surrounding fat and connective tissue. Therefore, all sonographic images in the aforementioned guide are accompanied by a schematic drawing to help make things clearer. In these instructions to clarify the dynamic changes of the different muscles in motion, each sonographic image in relaxation is accompanied by an image in maximum arbitrary contraction. The anatomic structures marked with numbers are named and explained underneath the appropriate images.

A similar detailed instruction with ultrasound and schematic pictures was published by Wu in 2022, discussing potential clinical relevance for every muscle [3].

Therefore, for a surgeon starting US of the face, reading both publications should be useful to acquire high-quality quantitative data for scientific research and evidence-based medicine [4–8].

Anyway, similar to photos or videos, ultrasound for assessing facial function and deficits can only quantify some aspects. Therefore, the gold standard should be a multimodal assessment using not only imaging and/or electrophysiological techniques, but also patient and expert related outcome measures and ideally (but nearly never used) ratings of lay persons.

Author Contributions: Conceptualization, O.G.-L.; writing—original draft preparation, G.F.V.; writing—review and editing, C.N. and R.Y.K.; funding acquisition, G.F.V. and O.G.-L. All authors have read and agreed to the published version of the manuscript.

Citation: Nduka, C.; Kannan, R.Y.; Volk, G.F.; Guntinas-Lichius, O. Comment on Kehrer et al. Using High-Resolution Ultrasound to Assess Post-Facial Paralysis Synkinesis—Machine Settings and Technical Aspects for Facial Surgeons. *Diagnostics* 2022, 12, 1650. *Diagnostics* 2022, 12, 2431. https://doi.org/10.3390/diagnostics12102431

Academic Editor: Hyung-kwon Byeon

Received: 13 July 2022
Accepted: 5 September 2022
Published: 8 October 2022

Publisher's Note: MDPI stays neutral with regard to jurisdictional claims in published maps and institutional affiliations.

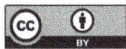

Copyright: © 2022 by the authors. Licensee MDPI, Basel, Switzerland. This article is an open access article distributed under the terms and conditions of the Creative Commons Attribution (CC BY) license (https://creativecommons.org/licenses/by/4.0/).

Funding: The APC was funded by Deutsche Gesellschaft für Ultraschall in der Medizin: Comparison of Ultrasound to Quantify the Effect of Surface Electrostimulation of Denervated Facial Muscles with MRI, 3D-Videos, and Expert Ratings.

Conflicts of Interest: The authors declare no conflict of interest.

References

1. Kehrer, A.; Ruewe, M.; Platz Batista da Silva, N.; Lonic, D.; Heidekrueger, P.I.; Knoedler, S.; Jung, E.M.; Prantl, L.; Knoedler, L. Using High-Resolution Ultrasound to Assess Post-Facial Paralysis Synkinesis—Machine Settings and Technical Aspects for Facial Surgeons. *Diagnostics* **2022**, *12*, 1650. [CrossRef] [PubMed]
2. Azizzadeh, B.; Nduka, C. (Eds.) Appendix—Instructions for Sonography of the Mimic Musculature. In *Management of Post-Facial Paralysis Synkinesis*; Elsevier: Amsterdam, The Netherlands, 2022; pp. 109–133, ISBN 9780323673310. Available online: https://www.sciencedirect.com/science/article/pii/B9780323673310150018 (accessed on 6 September 2022). [CrossRef]
3. Wu, W.-T.; Chang, K.-V.; Chang, H.-C.; Chen, L.-R.; Kuan, C.-H.; Kao, J.-T.; Wei, L.-Y.; Chen, Y.-J.; Han, D.-S.; Özçakar, L. Ultrasound Imaging of the Facial Muscles and Relevance with Botulinum Toxin Injections: A Pictorial Essay and Narrative Review. *Toxins* **2022**, *14*, 101. [CrossRef] [PubMed]
4. Sauer, M.; Guntinas-Lichius, O.; Volk, G.F. Ultrasound echomyography of facial muscles in diagnosis and follow-up of facial palsy in children. *Eur. J. Paediatr. Neurol.* **2016**, *20*, 666–670. [CrossRef] [PubMed]
5. Meiser, V.C.; Kreysa, H.; Guntinas-Lichius, O.; Volk, G.F. Comparison of in-plane and out-of-plane needle insertion with vs. without needle guidance. *Eur. Arch. Otorhinolaryngol.* **2016**, *273*, 2697–2705. [CrossRef] [PubMed]
6. Volk, G.F.; Leier, C.; Guntinas-Lichius, O. Correlation between electromyography and quantitative ultrasonography of facial muscles in patients with facial palsy. *Muscle Nerve* **2016**, *53*, 755–761. [CrossRef] [PubMed]
7. Volk, G.F.; Pohlmann, M.; Finkensieper, M.; Chalmers, H.J.; Guntinas-Lichius, O. 3D-Ultrasonography for evaluation of facial muscles in patients with chronic facial palsy or defective healing: A pilot study. *BMC Ear Nose Throat Disord.* **2014**, *14*, 4. [CrossRef] [PubMed]
8. Volk, G.F.; Sauer, M.; Pohlmann, M.; Guntinas-Lichius, O. Reference values for dynamic facial muscle ultrasonography in adults. *Muscle Nerve* **2014**, *50*, 348–357. [CrossRef] [PubMed]

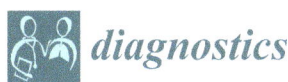

Reply

Reply to Nduka et al. Comment on "Kehrer et al. Using High-Resolution Ultrasound to Assess Post-Facial Paralysis Synkinesis—Machine Settings and Technical Aspects for Facial Surgeons. *Diagnostics* 2022, *12*, 1650"

Andreas Kehrer, Lukas Prantl, Samuel Knoedler and Leonard Knoedler *

Department of Plastic, Hand and Reconstructive Surgery, University Hospital Regensburg, 93053 Regensburg, Germany
* Correspondence: leonard.knoedler@stud.uni-regensburg.de; Tel.: +49-151-4482-4958

Citation: Kehrer, A.; Prantl, L.; Knoedler, S.; Knoedler, L. Reply to Nduka et al. Comment on "Kehrer et al. Using High-Resolution Ultrasound to Assess Post-Facial Paralysis Synkinesis—Machine Settings and Technical Aspects for Facial Surgeons. *Diagnostics* 2022, *12*, 1650". *Diagnostics* **2022**, *12*, 2432. https://doi.org/10.3390/diagnostics12102432

Academic Editor: Hyung-kwon Byeon

Received: 18 September 2022
Accepted: 29 September 2022
Published: 8 October 2022

Publisher's Note: MDPI stays neutral with regard to jurisdictional claims in published maps and institutional affiliations.

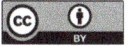

Copyright: © 2022 by the authors. Licensee MDPI, Basel, Switzerland. This article is an open access article distributed under the terms and conditions of the Creative Commons Attribution (CC BY) license (https://creativecommons.org/licenses/by/4.0/).

We thank Dr. Nduka et al. for this interesting article [1]. We very much enjoyed reading the detailed Instructions for Sonography of the Mimic Musculature [2]. We found the schematic, yet practice-orientated drawings helpful for visualizing the complex facial anatomical relationships and different planes. We see our structured working protocol as add-on to their work [3].

Together with other advancements in clinical facial palsy (FP) diagnostics and basic scientific translational efforts, such as automated grading systems or axon quantification, high-resolution ultrasound (HRUS) enlarges the FP surgeon's arsenal and understanding of FP disease [4–9].

Reading both publications, FP surgeons with basic levels of knowledge of facial HRUS may enhance their clinical workflow and refine their diagnostic setting in FP patients. Such an evidence-based approach might promote FP patient care, scientific data acquisition, and cost-effectiveness.

In future studies, the combination of facial HRUS and machine learning should explore the feasibility of automatizing this diagnostic step. Overall, facial HRUS represents a promising research field for both basic and clinical studies, and we are looking forward to future developments in facial HRUS.

Author Contributions: Investigation, A.K. and L.K.; writing—original draft preparation, A.K. and L.K.; writing—review and editing, L.P. and S.K. All authors have read and agreed to the published version of the manuscript.

Funding: This research received no external funding.

Conflicts of Interest: The authors declare no conflict of interest.

References

1. Nduka, C.; Kannan, R.Y.; Volk, G.F.; Guntinas-Lichius, O. Comment on Kehrer et al. Using High-Resolution Ultrasound to Assess Post-Facial Paralysis Synkinesis—Machine Settings and Technical Aspects for Facial Surgeons. *Diagnostics* 2022, *12*, 1650. *Diagnostics* **2022**, *12*, 2431. [CrossRef]
2. Azizzadeh, B.; Nduka, C. (Eds.) Appendix—Instructions for sonography of the mimic musculature. In *Management of Post-Facial Paralysis Synkinesis*; Elsevier: Amsterdam, The Netherlands, 2022; pp. 109–133.
3. Kehrer, A.; Ruewe, M.; da Silva, N.P.B.; Lonic, D.; Heidekrueger, P.I.; Knoedler, S.; Jung, E.M.; Prantl, L.; Knoedler, L. Using High-Resolution Ultrasound to Assess Post-Facial Paralysis Synkinesis—Machine Settings and Technical Aspects for Facial Surgeons. *Diagnostics* **2022**, *12*, 1650. [CrossRef] [PubMed]
4. Engelmann, S.; Ruewe, M.; Geis, S.; Taeger, C.D.; Kehrer, M.; Tamm, E.R.; Bleys, R.L.A.; Zeman, F.; Prantl, L.; Kehrer, A. Rapid and Precise Semi-Automatic Axon Quantification in Human Peripheral Nerves. *Sci. Rep.* **2020**, *10*, 1935. [CrossRef] [PubMed]
5. Ruewe, M.; Engelmann, S.; Huang, C.W.; Klein, S.M.; Anker, A.M.; Lamby, P.; Bleys, R.L.A.W.; Tamm, E.R.; Prantl, L.; Kehrer, A. Microanatomy of the Frontal Branch of the Facial Nerve: The Role of Nerve Caliber and Axonal Capacity. *Plast. Reconstr. Surg.* **2021**, *148*, 1357–1365. [CrossRef] [PubMed]
6. Kehrer, A.; Ruewe, M.; Engelmann, S.; Anker, A.; Taeger, C.; Geis, S.; Prantl, L. From bench-to-bedside: Implications for facial reanimation surgery gained from axonal load quantification and nerve morphometry of a cadaver study in 106 facial halves. In Proceedings of the Annual Meeting of the American Society for Reconstructive Microsurgery, Fort Lauderdale, FL, USA, 10–14 January 2020.
7. Kehrer, A.; Engelmann, S.; Ruewe, M.; Geis, S.; Taeger, C.; Kehrer, M.; Prantl, L.; Tamm, E.; Bleys, R.R.; Mandlik, V. Anatomical study of the zygomatic and buccal branches of the facial nerve: Application to facial reanimation procedures. *Clin. Anat.* **2019**, *32*, 480–488. [CrossRef] [PubMed]
8. Sommerauer, L.; Engelmann, S.; Ruewe, M.; Anker, A.; Prantl, L.; Kehrer, A. Effects of electrostimulation therapy in facial nerve palsy. *Arch. Plast. Surg.* **2021**, *48*, 278–281. [CrossRef] [PubMed]
9. Kehrer, A.; Mandlik, V.; Taeger, C.; Geis, S.; Prantl, L.; Jung, E.-M. Postoperative control of functional muscle flaps for facial palsy reconstruction: Ultrasound guided tissue monitoring using contrast enhanced ultrasound (CEUS) and ultrasound elastography. *Clin. Hemorheol. Microcirc.* **2017**, *67*, 435–444. [CrossRef] [PubMed]

MDPI
St. Alban-Anlage 66
4052 Basel
Switzerland
www.mdpi.com

Diagnostics Editorial Office
E-mail: diagnostics@mdpi.com
www.mdpi.com/journal/diagnostics

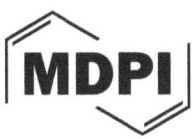

Disclaimer/Publisher's Note: The statements, opinions and data contained in all publications are solely those of the individual author(s) and contributor(s) and not of MDPI and/or the editor(s). MDPI and/or the editor(s) disclaim responsibility for any injury to people or property resulting from any ideas, methods, instructions or products referred to in the content.

www.ingramcontent.com/pod-product-compliance
Lightning Source LLC
LaVergne TN
LVHW070608100526
838202LV00012B/598